SIMPLE STEPS...COSTLY CHOICES

A Guide to Inner Peace

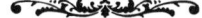

Other Books by the Author

By Streams of Water

On Earth As It Is...
Discovering God's Grace in the Ordinary

SIMPLE STEPS...COSTLY CHOICES

A Guide to Inner Peace

Bob Lively

With Foreword by Dr. Gerald Man

Riverbend Press
Austin, Texas

Copyright © 1995 by Robert Lively

All rights reserved. No part of this book may be reproduced or utilized in any form or by any means, electronic or mechanical, including photocopying, recording or by any information storage and retrieval system, without permission in writing from the publisher. Inquiries should be addressed to:

Permissions Department
Riverbend Press
4214 Capital of Texas Hwy.
Austin, Texas 78746

Library of Congress Cataloging-in-Publication Data
Lively, Robert

Simple Steps...Costly Choices: A Guide to Inner Peace

Includes bibliographical references.

ISBN 0-9647272-4-2 $14.95

1. Recovery   I. Title
2. 12-Steps
3. Grace

95-74832   1995

9 8 7 6 5 4 3 2 1

Printed in the United States of America at Austin, Texas

Dedicated to the memory of

William Jesse Lively,

Who taught me what grace looks like.

Acknowledgments

The writing of acknowledgments is, at best, a risky enterprise in that invariably someone gets overlooked. This is my third book, and as careful as I have been with the past two acknowledgment pages I have written, I have omitted names that should have been, and by all rights, needed to be included.

Be that as it may, I hereby humbly submit a symbolic page, and nothing more than that, that lists the names of a few of the literally scores of folks who made this publication possible.

I thank Mr. Stan Cobbs for his efforts in securing a cozy writing cabin at Presbyterian Mo-Ranch Assembly during a cold winter month when a herd of white tail deer, a persistent Cooper's hawk, a flock of wild turkeys and one tenacious house cat and I dwelled together in both seclusion and harmony in the Texas Hill Country.

I thank Dr. Gerald Mann, not only for the Foreword he provided for this book, but also for the necessary permission that afforded me the opportunity to retreat long enough from the world to bring this book idea to fruition.

I wish to thank Ms. Kathy Bork, a long-time friend, for her professional editorial expertise, and I also offer profound thanks to Ms. Melondie Gentry for her excellent proofreading skills.

I further wish to thank the newly founded Riverbend Press which honored me by agreeing to make this small book its initial publication. In the specific context of this effort, I thank Mr. Preston Tyree, Ms. Charla Long, Ms. Sharon Wharton, and my trusted colleague and friend, the Reverend Mike Rinehart.

Further, I wish to thank Ms. Wendy Lawrence for her editorial assistance and my most capable colleague and good friend, the Reverend Dr. Gordon Smith for his willingness to "cover" for me so effectively while I was away from the office writing this book.

I give further thanks to my family for a lifetime of love, to the congregation of Riverbend Church for their consistent emotional support, and to those who believed in me even when others turned away. Most of all, I give thanks to God for the gift of my suffering so that through it I could come to know grace.

I sought the Lord, and he answered me, and delivered me from all of my fears.

Psalm 34: 4 Revised Standard Version

The Twelve Steps to Inner Peace

Step 1: I admit I am powerless over _____, and that my life has become unmanageable.

Step 2: I believe that a power (I say God as revealed in Jesus Christ) greater than me can restore me to sanity.

Step 3: I turn my will and my life over to the care of God as I understand God.

Step 4: I make a fearless moral inventory of myself.

Step 5: I admit to God the exact nature of my wrongs.

Step 6: I am entirely ready to have God remove all these defects of my character.

Step 7: I humbly ask God to remove my shortcomings.

Step 8: I make a list of those persons I have harmed, and I prepare myself to make amends to them all.

Step 9: I make direct amends to such people wherever possible, except when to do so would injure them or others.

Step 10: I continue to take personal inventory and when I am wrong, I promptly admit it.

Step 11: I seek through prayer and meditation to improve my conscious contact with God, as I understand God, praying only for knowledge of God's will for me and for the power to carry it out.

Step 12: Through my own spiritual awakening, I carry this message to others, and practice these principles in all my affairs.

Contents

Foreword: by Dr. Gerald Mann xi

Introduction xiii

Chapter 1: 1

    I admit I am powerless over _____, and that my life has become unmanageable.

Chapter 2: 19

    I believe that a power (I say God as revealed in Jesus Christ) greater than me can restore me to sanity.

Chapter 3: 37

    I turn my will and my life over to the care of God as I understand God.

Chapter 4: 55

    I make a fearless moral inventory of myself.

Chapter 5: 69

    I admit to God the exact nature of my wrongs.

Chapter 6: 85

    I am entirely ready to have God remove all these defects of my character.

Chapter 7: 101

    I humbly ask God to remove my shortcomings.

Chapter 8: 119

    I make a list of those persons I have harmed, and I prepare myself to make amends to them all.

Chapter 9: 147

    I make direct amends to such people wherever possible, except when to do so would injure them or others.

Chapter 10: 153

    I continue to take personal inventory and when I am wrong, I promptly admit it.

Chapter 11: 169

    I seek through prayer and meditation to improve my conscious contact with God, as I understand God, praying only for knowledge of God's will for me and for the power to carry it out.

Chapter 12: 185

    Through my own spiritual awakening, I carry this message to others, and practice these principles in all my affairs.

Bibliography 193

Foreword

Fifteen years ago I helped found a church with one simple goal: to reach people no one else could reach or wanted to reach. Being from a Baptist background, I began by searching for disenfranchised Baptists.

Who were the Baptist drop outs and cast-offs in our community? Among the most obvious were Baptists with drinking problems. No church bothered with them. There were no ecclesiastical competitors in the field.

But there was a competitor which was more formidable than any church when it came to affecting real spiritual transformation in the lives of people. This "foe" would change my life as well. It would teach me more about what it means to be the church than anything I had learned in the halls of religious academia or in twenty years of pastoring.

The ingenious Twelve Step program of recovery changes people from the inside out. In a world which loves to describe a problem, the Twelve Step program *prescribes* a cure for the deepest human addictions. It enables people to experience conversion, both the psychological and the spiritual kind.

And, as I was to discover, we are all addicted to something. It is the human condition, pure and simple. Addiction is simply another way of describing "Original Sin."

The Twelve Steps are simply another way of communicating and putting into practice the Good News which frees people from their enslavements. I call the Program, "The Gospel in Drag."

The founders of Alcoholics Anonymous had to remove most of the religious language from the Steps in order to accommodate sick people who couldn't handle "another sermon."

All of the biblical ingredients of spiritual conversion are contained in the Twelve Steps:
- Confession of our helpless condition;
- Repentance—turning from destructive patterns;
- Faith—entrusting the management of our destiny to a Higher Power;
- Community—the supportive and corrective environment offered by the church;
- Santification—a never ending working and re-working of the recovering steps;
- Works & faith—taking constant moral inventory;
- Sharing—our spiritual experiences with others; and

- Forgiveness—acceptance without judging those who slip.

I now have a "church full" of Twelve Steppers. I call them "The Kingdom's Commandos." God is sending Twelve Steppers under cover to infiltrate churches today. Their mission is to teach us what churching is all about.

I'll take all of them I can get. Often, Twelve Steppers tell me they don't need the church. I tell them they're probably correct, but the church surely does need them, especially if its mission is to heal sick souls.

For years I've thought of writing a book which translates the Twelve Steps back into the religious and psychological language from which they sprung. I envisioned a book for people who were addicted to something besides alcohol or other drugs, and therefore couldn't resonate to the A. A. jargon. I was thinking of a "blend" of biblical, psychological, and therapeutic categories which would click with the modern mind.

It was this kind of "re-translation" that revolutionized my life and led to the birth of the healing church I serve in Austin, Texas.

I'm addicted to several things over which I have no power at all. Success is one. I'm a child who craves the spotlight. My infantile need for adulation is insatiable. Fixing everyone and everything is another. I have no power over my addiction to make the world stop and go at my command.

But these addictions have been controlled and redeemed—as of today—by Another. "Higher Power," "God," "Yahweh." —He is called by many names. I call Him "Grace." He won't give up on me, even though I give up on him regularly.

Anyway, I never wrote the book, for several reasons. Perhaps the main one is that God wanted Bob Lively to write it.

This book certainly is what I had in mind: The Twelve Steps re-translated into a biblical, spiritual, and psychological language for the modern mind, and made applicable to any and all of our addictions.

Bob's book, in my opinion, captures the best of the revelations of God to the human sciences, to theology, and to everyday experience. If you know you have "the disease" which we all share in common, you can make the first step toward wholeness. Read on.

Dr. Gerald Mann
Austin, Texas 1995

Introduction

I am addicted to fear. I am not powerless over alcohol. I am not addicted to any drug. In fact, I've never ingested an illegal drug in my life. Still, I have become convinced that I have the same disease as an alcoholic or drug addict. Some folks call it alcoholism; I most often call it "the disease."

For years I honestly did not know that I had a disease. Oh, I had suffered from the standard childhood illnesses—mumps, chicken pox, measles—which are as much a part of human development as puberty and the awkwardness that invariably attends adolescence. But I no more recognized a disease dwelling deep in my soul than a crowing rooster possesses insight into the existential meaning of his early-morning signal to a community of sleepy citizens.

I lived, and more or less coped, with the symptoms of this insidious disease, but, in truth, I never named it, much less treated the thing. Its symbols are what those who inhabit the world of "mental health" would term "symptoms."

And what were these symptoms? The garden-variety stuff right out of the mental health world's Bible, the *DSM IV*: depression, what the psychiatrists term "a dysthymic disorder." In lay terms, such a depression is a kind of low-grade, long-term malaise that has a way of gnawing at the soul the way rust slowly chews on good metal.

In addition, I was diagnosed with an amorphous anxiety disorder that usually presented itself as what, again employing clinical language, would best be termed a "social phobia." And what is my social phobia? In simplest terms, I am terrified of standing before groups, even small groups, and presenting any kind of material. In short, I have a fear (terror is more descriptive) of public speaking.

Social phobia is not a wonderful disorder to haul around when one has decided or, as in my case, has felt "called" to enter a profession where preaching, teaching, and officiating on occasions of great formality, such as weddings, baptisms, and funerals, are regular duties.

Anxiety and depression were not only my symptoms of the disease of fear addiction, they became my daily companions, as well. They ate at me. They haunted me. In truth, they controlled me.

My childhood was, and remains in my perception, an idyllic existence where, from the "git go," as I often heard any kind of beginning described in the Piney Woods of East Texas, I recognized beyond the shadow of any doubt that I was loved and accepted by spiritually mature parents and three loving, mischievous brothers.

How, then, did I contract this disease? I do not possess any more insight into that today than when I set out on the arduous journey into my soul two decades ago. I simply do not know. But you must understand that this question is a *"Why?"* question, and I have come to believe that most if not all such questions are irrelevant to healing.

The relevant question is always *"What?" What* am I learning from these symptoms or symbols that have come to torment me? And what must I do to heed their message? These are the relevant questions that shepherd me toward genuine healing.

In my experience over the past decade as a pastoral counselor, I have come to view *Why* questions as an intellectual vortex into which our psychic and emotional energy is too often sucked. We end up exhausted from chasing solutions to questions we can't answer. Therefore, I now concentrate on discovering the *Whats* in my life. More often than not, it is those *What* questions that have put me on the path to the truth.

In the context of our healing, the truth is all that really matters. If this book is to be helpful to anyone, it must be the truth. And the truth is that I have suffered for most, if not all, of my life with two disorders, mild depression and fear of public speaking, which I have come to regard as symptoms of the disease.

One additional question begging for an honest response regards what other characterological disorders underlie the more obvious dysthymic disorder (mild depression) and the social phobia disorder (fear of public speaking). As best as I can discern, I do not possess a strongly disordered character. I am, without question, passive and, all too often, passive-aggressive. I am narcissistic, and, if I am not careful, I can easily lapse into overdependence on other human beings, whom I "seduce" emotionally into rescuing me. In my less-healthy moments, and when I am not consciously working the principles of the 12 Steps, I can quite easily lapse into sick behaviors that encourage others to think for me and even to feel for me.

Today, I am satisfied that I am what would most likely be termed, again employing the common parlance of the mental health world, a "healthy neurotic" rather than the possessor of a full-blown personality disorder.

Introduction

I am far more demanding of myself than I have ever been of other folks.

Such a differentiation is the criterion most often marking the boundary between neurosis and character disorders. Neurotics tend to be at war with themselves. Such tension describes me accurately. Personality-disordered people, on the other hand, tend to be at war with the world in either an aggressive mode or in driving the rest of us crazy with sick thinking and unhealthy behaviors.

I first became aware of my fear addiction when its symptoms presented themselves during my brief stint in Lyndon Johnson's ill-conceived and, in retrospect, wholly ineffectual War on Poverty. To sidestep the draft and thereby to avoid participating in another kind of war in which I could not bring myself to fight, I "enlisted" in one of VISTA's specialized branches, the National Teacher Corps.

The idea of the Teacher Corps seemed noble enough on paper, and to my naïve mind, it appeared a sound alternative to traveling halfway across the globe to do battle with a people against whom I could not find one solid reason to fight. Therefore, I cast my lot with the Teacher Corps in that it squared with my budding wish to do battle with ignorance rather than to wage war on other human beings.

I was assigned to the village of Lexington, Texas, approximately fifty miles from the state capital, Austin. My assignment was as simple as it was challenging: I was to teach reading, history, or whatever else I could help with, to students who, in the main, were what we termed back then the "culturally deprived."

In the early afternoon of Valentine's Day of 1969, I was standing before a tiny class of eighth graders and was lecturing them, in my best high-toned, pseudo-intellectual demeanor, on the American Civil War's impact on our culture.

Suddenly, from out of nowhere, a sense of terror raced through my consciousness. The physical symptoms that followed were more frightening than anything I had ever experienced. I could no longer speak. I literally could not form words. I suppose I had heard of the phenomenon, but I had never in my wildest imagination believed that such a thing could happen to me.

My heart began to pound. I was certain that I was experiencing a coronary. My palms sweated, and so much perspiration burst from my forehead that it must have appeared to those startled students that their still-wet-behind-the-ears twenty-two-year-old teacher had gone stark raving mad.

I motioned to a colleague, who immediately rose from her desk and ran to me. I managed to utter, "I am sick . . . Please take the class. I must be coming down with something."

I abandoned the classroom and stumbled through the front door of the small school and into the cold drizzle of that mid-February afternoon. I remember the call of a crow on the far side of a muddy pasture. The sound soothed me as it momentarily returned me to the familiar moorings of my spiritual home, the East Texas Piney Woods.

I most recall an overwhelming sense of longing to die. I had never before even thought in those terms, but trembling in the muddy ruts of the road leading to the fifty-dollar-a-month rent house I called home, I suddenly wanted to die.

It was an odd kind of ideation in that I really was in no way suicidal. I was, I now realize, suffering from such humiliation that I could see no way that I might continue the journey toward healthy adult maturation. No, I simply thought it better that I lie down in the cold February mud and die.

I dropped to my knees and dug my fingernails into the mud. I cried out, but only a curious crow heard my agony.

I cried out a second time, but again there was no answer, not even from the crow. My first lucid thought was that I was experiencing the trauma and travail that had beset the apostle Paul on the road to Damascus. But I still possessed enough clarity to realize that these ruts did not lead to Damascus. No, this unpaved road pointed only in the direction of denial, "workaholism," depression, and fear.

My world after that experience might best be described as upside-down. I would later come to call the episode "an acute anxiety attack," but at the time, I only knew never to allow myself to reflect upon the incident. With every fiber of my being I sought to deny it. And never once did I even consider sharing the magnitude of my terror with anyone, lest they think I might consider myself insane.

I left the Teacher Corps a year early so that I might enroll at a small Presbyterian seminary. On the first day of orientation, I heard words that sent chills down my spine.

The director of admissions grinned wider than a mule chewing prickly pear and announced, "Tomorrow you will have administered to you the MMPI." A young man sitting to my right raised his hand and inquired as to the meaning underlying the acronym. The director explained that MMPI stood for Minnesota Multiphase Personality Inventory.

I immediately considered withdrawal from seminary, but I knew that such a decision could prove costly, if not altogether dangerous. The Vietnam War was raging at its highest pitch. I had resigned from the Teacher Corps, and I literally had no viable alternatives. It was either endure the seminary-imposed MMPI or enlist in the army and wage battle in violation of what I was fast coming to recognize were my most sacred values. I gave limited consideration to escaping to Canada, where other young men who had failed to achieve the status of conscientious objector had fled, and for a few hours I even pondered what it would mean for me go to prison as a political prisoner for my unwillingness to participate in the violence of Southeast Asia.

Remaining in the seminary and taking the MMPI seemed, by far, the best but not, for me, the least frightening option. I was now convinced that I was absolutely crazy. I had learned to hide it, although what had for the whole of my short lifetime given me great joy—dining out, attending worship regularly, speaking persuasively, even passionately, before large groups, and leaving the security of home for wild adventures to exotic places—had all become objects of dread or the subject of nightmares. I remember myself as relaxed and somewhat confident amidst the givens of adolescent awkwardness, but I had turned overnight into a terrified young man.

I believed that I could not afford for anyone to know my secret; therefore, I began plotting how to avoid taking the test. No sound idea presented itself, so at the appointed hour I showed up with the rest of that entering class. With a stubby, chewed-up No. 2 pencil, I answered as honestly as I knew how the five hundred true and false questions.

I turned in the exam and immediately lit upon a second idea. I decided that I would not show up for the evaluation with the psychiatrist assigned by the seminary to visit with each prospective student regarding the test's results. I was on the threshold of learning how to cope at the seminary, and I figured that I might be able to bluff my way through the first semester. I suppose I convinced myself to hope against hope that somehow the Vietnam War might end and that I could return to some kind of civilian endeavor where I would not be "found out" through such demonic devices as the MMPI.

The director of admissions informed me of what I already knew, that I had missed my appointment with the psychiatrist. With far more politeness than I deserved, he further informed me that if I did not visit with the doctor, I would not be permitted to continue my studies at the seminary.

My back was now shoved against the proverbial wall. I do not believe I had ever been so frightened as I was on that Tuesday afternoon when I finally drove to the psychiatrist's office. Much to my dismay and embarrassment, I discovered that the wife of one of my classmates was the receptionist.

She pretended not to know me, and for that small favor I was more than a little grateful. But still I was terrified as I shuffled through the worn pages of a *Life Magazine*. Within minutes, my new friend's wife motioned for me to enter a room, where I was greeted by a well-groomed man who was, surprisingly, not much older than I.

He reclined in a large overstuffed leather chair while I, perched on the edge of an obviously expensive sofa, waited for the bad news. He smiled and reported to me that basically I was healthy, but that I did seem to suffer from anxiety and depression. He inquired regarding my experience with anxiety attacks and the like. Of course, I wagged my head in the direction of "No."

He stood and, to my shock, failed to pronounce me "insane." He did recommend, however, that I seek some kind of therapy somewhere. I had never really heard the word before in the context of what little I knew about mental health, but in some strange way, the invitation brought to my awareness a new sense of relief.

I recall driving back to the seminary while fighting hard against the wave of tears that, at least in my own frightened thoughts, now threatened to drown me. One thought rolled over and over again in my mind: "Maybe I am not crazy. Maybe what has happened to me is, after all, explainable and, more than that, even treatable."

For the first time in six months I discovered some small measure of hope. I called the psychiatrist's office the next morning and scheduled a second appointment. I informed my friend's wife that I planned to pursue "therapy."

I began a string of half-hour sessions with the doctor who had interpreted my test. He seemed neither interested in me as a person nor particularly calloused. He listened, hummed occasionally, cleared his throat often, and at least once every session offered what I regarded to be a genuinely encouraging insight or remark.

At the end of the initial session he prescribed a new drug—Valium. By God's grace, and only by that, I did not become addicted to it. But I did use it off and on for the remainder of that first semester. By Christmas the psychiatrist pronounced me "better." We shook hands, I waved goodbye to his receptionist, and I was more than satisfied that I was now "fixed." I never refilled my prescription.

The next two years convinced me that I had been cured. Hard work was followed by achievement and even some small measure of recognition. I was elected president of the student body and I went on to graduate with honors.

In some circuitous way I equated my newfound mental health with achievement. The formula was, for me, as simple as it was erroneous: achieve to the point of being recognized by others and then you will become acceptable even to yourself. Hard work, discipline, and accomplishment were, for me, the single path to relief from the unsettling conviction that I might be "unacceptable."

In theological terms, my more unconscious than conscious soteriological formula went like this: God demands perfection; therefore I *must* in all things be perfect; I *should* always drive myself without even a hint of mercy; I *must*, whatever the personal cost, get myself recognized. Grace, what little I knew of it, thus became equated with a virulent narcissism.

And as ludicrous as it sounds today, I truly believed that my salvation lay in fame. I was convinced that if I could just get "famous," whatever that meant, I would finally be okay in that I would then finally accept myself. Therefore, for me, the path to the kingdom of God was marked with an austere signpost that directed me to places like Righteous Zeal, Harsh Discipline, Obedience, Boundless Shame, Mindless Determination, and Abject Terror. I was convinced that nothing else in this world could save me from my despair except daily herculean effort.

The more I scared myself with such nonsense, the harder I worked. On one level, the scheme seemed to work. I was more surprised than anyone regarding what I was able to accomplish under the noble, even pious, rubric of "doing ministry."

But the fact is that the symbols did not dissipate. The symptoms of dysthymic disorder and social phobia continued unabated. The harder I worked, the more miserable I became.

I was in a bind in which many of us find ourselves. My life looked pretty good on the surface: I was an accomplished, respected, even somewhat sought-after young professional. I was absolutely miserable, however, but terrified to admit it, even to myself. Denial became, for me, a way of life.

Therefore, I sought help. I figured that there had to be more to this therapy business than stroking one's chin, "oohing and ahhing" at appropriate interludes, and prescribing medicine. My first stop was with a clergyman who had returned to graduate school to earn counseling credentials. He was and is a kind, insightful man, but I see now that he had been trained in the *Why* questions. Consequently, his probing was, in the main, ineffectual.

I pretended to feel better because I did not want to injure this man's ego. I shook his hand as he pronounced me "cured." I returned to my vision of "saving Dallas" (such ideation provides a glimpse into the depth of my narcissism) and in the ensuing years, my symbols (symptoms) became more pronounced than ever.

One December morning a woman I respected asked me how I would spend six hundred dollars that had been donated to the church with the stipulation that I spend them on me. "Easy," I blurted. "I would go buy me six efficacious 'therapy' hours." I still had no more idea than a billy goat what this thing called "therapy" was about. But if I was certain of anything, it was this—six hundred dollars would, no doubt, purchase me six high-dollar sessions with one of Dallas' best.

I was referred to a psychologist who turned out to be one of the most bizarre characters I have ever encountered. I suppose I did not mind wasting someone else's money; therefore, I enjoyed this man's antics more than I permitted him to be of any real help.

As my granddaddy used to say on our farm, this man was crazy as a "Betsy bug," whatever a "Betsy bug" is. When his telephone would ring, which was often in the midst of our counseling sessions, he would jump up and answer it, leaving me alone to ponder whatever part of my soul I had just unfurled. I could easily discern, because he held his telephone conversations not six feet from my place on his exquisite sofa, that most of what he talked about could comfortably fall under the category of chit-chat.

Here I was paying this man one hundred of someone else's dollars an hour to hear him visit with his buddies about deer hunting. Of course, I was far too passive and much too impressed by both his credentials and his standing in the community to confront him. After four sessions, I pronounced myself "healed," shook the man's hand, and invited him to keep the remaining two hundred of someone else's hard-earned dollars.

I gave up on this thing called therapy. I figured that at best it was one caring human being listening to and loving another; at its worst, it was pat formulas, smoke and mirrors.

For reasons that I am now certain had far more to do with the unconscious search for my own healing than with anything conscious, in 1985, after what could only be described as a successful, though secretly painful, ten-year stint in the parish, I applied for a position as a full-time resident in a training program accredited by the American Association of Pastoral Counselors. I was accepted.

For two wonderful, arduous, and confusing years, I struggled to learn to become what deep down I was convinced did not exist, namely, a therapist. I applied myself, just as I had done in college and seminary, and the results were the same. I was respected by my colleagues and, after only a short time in the program, I was informed rather consistently that I im-

Introduction

pressed those who sought to train me. All of this meant only one thing—I was once again desperately seeking acceptance.

It was in the context of this training that I was assigned to work with a gifted and dedicated counselor named Kathy who was running a group for "healthy neurotics," many of whom reported past issues with drug and alcohol abuse.

Rather routinely Kathy would launch into her own story of having "the disease" but without the symptoms of substance abuse. I questioned her claim. How, I asked myself, could anyone be an alcoholic and not be powerless in the face of alcohol? The concept made no more sense to me than the physics problems I had struggled with in college.

Of course, because I was seeking to impress (and therefore be accepted by) others, especially Kathy, I dared not pose the question out loud. I simply decided that if Kathy believed she had this disease, then such a conviction was acceptable to me. After all, it was her disease, not mine.

Call it grace. Call it divine intervention. Call it whatever you wish. (But I would not go so far as to term it any kind of full-fledged theophany.) The thought one evening arrived in my conscious mind like some boorish, uninvited old relative who comes to visit then refuses to leave. Its content was as simple as it was terrifying: Bob, you have the same disease that Kathy has described so eloquently for the past several months.

Perhaps I was placed by some divine coincidence in her presence so that I might finally bump into the truth about my own long-term suffering. I don't know about all of that. But if I am absolutely convinced of any truth about myself today, it is this: I have the same disease as the alcoholic or the drug addict. My addiction is fear.

I have been drunk once, on the night that I discovered that I would not be drafted. In fact, I got so drunk that I convinced myself that I spotted a porcupine high atop a Colorado lodge pole pine. I shimmied up the tree only to slip and then tumble to the ground. I awoke some time later, crawled to my car, and again, only by God's grace, made it to a ranch where I was employed at the time.

The next day I was required to ride a horse from sunup until dusk, and never again, not in close to thirty years, have I had more than one drink per day. Therefore, I can write with integrity that I am not powerless over alcohol.

I have never ingested any kind of illegal substance. I have never even smoked marijuana. But I remain convinced that I have the disease.

How can that be? In addressing that question, it is as tempting as jumping into a cold spring on an August afternoon to become entangled in the whys of this disease. I do not know why is the only answer I can offer. I do not know how it is that I came to have this disease, but I am certain that I do have it. In the popular parlance of the '90s, I have it big time!

The more I have studied this insidious disease, the more I have come to believe that for all of us who have the disease, our addiction has its roots in fear. From the time that we become conscious in childhood, we learn to be afraid of two realities: life and death. Consequently, as budding human beings we are thrust by circumstances woefully beyond our control into an arena where, like it or not, we are required to make a decision. We must accept and face our fears regarding the responsibilities that life foists upon us, or we must give in to death even while we are walking around and breathing.

This giving in to death does not mean, of course, that we die physically; it is more like a spiritual death in that we swap a conscious decision to step into our fear for an unconscious decision to allow our life to be controlled by it.

And it is this terrible, though often unconscious, decision to relinquish life to fear that sets us up for the disease. The disease leads us in the direction of defending against the fear by avoiding what I believe Jesus had in mind when he spoke two thousand years ago of "abundant life." Simply put, there can be no abundant life when fear controls our lives.

So, for whatever it is worth, my simple, but I hope not simplistic, definition of the disease is this: a human life governed by conscious and unconscious fear. It makes no real difference to this definition if the features of drug and alcohol dependency attend the disease in symptomatic forms. The disease remains the same—it is the human life governed by conscious and unconscious fear.

I have never claimed to be much of a scholar of anything, and I regard myself to be a student of even less. Nevertheless, I have a hunch that during the Jews' exile into that strange land known as Babylon, they became totally immersed in the culture. For good or ill, those folks from Palestine gained a radically new perspective of the world, which included, of course, a whole new language.

I am told that one term they carried back with them to Jerusalem was "Satan." In Babylon it meant simply "adversary." Theologically, that is precisely the way I view Satan today—as my adversary.

I have come to believe that the adversary for those of us with this disease is unbridled, denied, defended, and therefore unconscious, fear. My guess is that the ancients had a name for what drove a good man or woman to drink to such excess that he or she destroyed a perfectly good life. And that force is what they termed the Adversary, or Satan.

Introduction

All manner of theological implication in the Scripture points directly to the conviction that Satan is a transcendent being. That may well be true. There is certainly evidence in the headlines that greet us each morning at the breakfast table. I simply do not know about that.

My own theological view is somewhat different, however. I view God as both immanent (inside of each of us) and transcendent (beyond us). And I tend to perceive of the Adversary (Satan) as *only* immanent. For me, then, Satan is an internal force more than a transcendent power or being. Further, Satan is that adversary that longs to seduce me away from trusting God completely in every dimension of my life.

I could be as wrong as two left boots, as my granddaddy used to say. Of course, I do not ever wish to mislead anyone, but I honestly believe that what I term "soul-capturing and life-controlling fear" is what the ancients termed Satan, or the Adversary.

It was out of this conviction and in response to the healing that I have discovered in the 12 Steps that I decided to write this book. Let me be clear at the outset. *This book is not the truth.* Only God is the Truth. This book is nothing more than one recovering man's desire to be faithful to the program.

My friend and colleague Dr. Gerald Mann, senior pastor of Riverbend Church, stopped me on the church sidewalk on a gorgeous spring day recently. His question stunned me at first: "Bob, there really are more than 12 Steps, aren't there?" I remember thinking, "You could have fooled me. I thought the program consisted of 12 Steps."

I decided against interrupting a man I have come to know as brilliant. He continued, "No, there are in reality 12 million steps, because to make it work we have to do each step a million times."

He is exactly right. Therefore, let me be clear. This book is not my final Step. No, this modest work is my latest 12th Step, and there is a world of difference between working a final Step and doing the 12th Step. And where do I go as soon as I turn this manuscript over to the publisher? I return to Step 1, where I will admit again, just as I do every day, that I am powerless over my fear or over my adversary, Satan.

If you have read this far, you are most likely asking the question that is as common as fleas on a country dog's backside: "Will these 12 Steps work for what ails me?"

I don't know. But I have discovered amazing healing in these Steps. They have allowed me to discover a "therapist" who has helped me in ways I never expected. In fact, I have come to learn through this process that this "healer" knows far more about what I need than I do. The name of the physician, of course, is God. And through the discipline of these

Steps I have come to trust the healer, quite imperfectly, one day at a time.

And what has been the result? The answer to that is nothing less than miraculous. Where there was once a social phobia, I today savor speaking before large, on occasion, even massive audiences. Where there was depression, there are days of honest, down-to-earth joy. Where there was obsession and its first cousin, compulsion (workaholism), today there is inner peace and frequent laughter. Today I enjoy quiet evenings, time to write poetry no one will ever read, long nights of peaceful sleep, more time than ever for prayer, daily walks, and, most important, love.

Is my life perfect? Of course not. Does my life work? Yes, it does, when I stop attempting to *make* it work. Does the depression return? Occasionally, but it has never come back with the vengeance that was once its trademark. Am I still afraid? Of course. I still tremble some when I stand to perform a wedding or when I am interviewed on live radio. But I have learned to give my terror, as well as the rest of my life, to God one day at a time. And in the process, I have discovered that I am the heir to what Jesus promised when he spoke two thousand years ago of having an "abundant life."

My life is not perfect but, in truth, it is abundant. The glory goes to God and to the path to God that finally offered me genuine healing—the 12 Steps.

As the title of this book suggests, the Steps are quite simple, but they are in no way easy, not easy at all. If you are reading this book as a neophyte in the search for inner peace, expect the Steps to be difficult. That way you will not be disappointed. Allow me to say it again: the Steps are so simple that even a preliterate child could, at the minimal level necessary for efficacy, understand them. But these Steps are not easy.

So, if you take this journey toward wholeness and healing, expect to stumble and slip. You will. There is no shame in it. Every one of us who has sought to discover our healing on this path has been there and will, no doubt, continue our "slip-sliding" approach to God for as long as God grants us breath to breathe in the context of our own spiritual journey.

I invite you to read each of these Steps thoroughly prior to taking your first Step. Then, and only if you are ready to feel better and live the life of courage that genuine faith requires, take that first Step. Admit your powerlessness over whatever it is that grips your soul. And then get out of the way and permit one who is far more intelligent and far more insightful than you or I could ever be to have some small part of your life.

Do not turn over too much too fast. You will probably not be ready for that kind of trust and you may end up even more defeated than when you began. Turn over something relatively small, like an insignificant resentment or a mid-range stressor, such as the irritation you feel when your father-in-law launches into a sexist tirade. Or turn over the fear you feel when your adolescent drives off on what we once called a "car date." Begin with the small things and build from there.

You will make it. The path is not smooth, but it is the right path, and in my view, this is the only path along which genuine healing of the soul occurs.

Should you seek professional help while you are on this path? That, of course, is entirely up to you. If you do seek such counsel, inquire of the therapist regarding his or her view of the 12 Steps. If the therapist is comfortable with the 12 Steps and has no problem with your working them concurrently with your one-on-one or couples therapy, go ahead and enter into a therapeutic relationship. If, on the other hand, the therapist debunks the 12 Steps, I would recommend that you look elsewhere. There are many fine psychiatrists, social workers, psychologists, and certified pastoral counselors who are strong proponents of the 12 Steps and who may serve you well as a guide on this miraculous path toward healing.

I have one final anecdote to offer before we take our first Step together. Last winter I was participating in a recovery group in Austin on a particularly cold, drizzly day. We were well into the meeting when the door popped open and an attractive young woman entered the room. I had never laid eyes on her, but I discerned by the nods she received from the other members that she was apparently a friend to many in this group.

When it came time for her to speak, she said something like this: "For the whole of my life, I have been mistaken. I once believed that I was a human being struggling to have a spiritual experience. Today, however, I have come to recognize that all along I have been a spiritual being struggling to have a human experience."

May a similar awakening come to you. My prayer is that this small book might help you along the path to wholeness and inner peace.

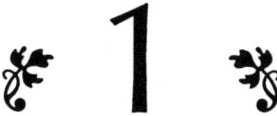

> When he saw the crowds, he had compassion for them, because they were harassed and helpless, like sheep without a shepherd.
>
> Matthew 9:36 RSV

Step 1 :   I admit I am powerless over _____, and that my life has become unmanageable.

Following the first year of my seminary training, I was mandated by the requirements for ordination in the Presbyterian Church U.S. (The Southern Presbyterian Church) to sit for fifteen hours of psychological tests with a woman in Dallas who had a reputation for scaring the spit out of candidates for the ministry.

In that I had been "cured" by the psychiatrist to whom I referred in the introduction, I was not nearly so anxious when I entered this woman's plush Dallas office as I might have been. In fact, I never even laid eyes on this terror until I returned the following week to have my scores interpreted.

I will never forget her icy critique of me and what she judged to be my "fitness for ministry." First she said, "You are not gay."

I recall grinning and working to reduce the obvious tension by offering some disarmingly folksy, but inane, response like, "Well, ma'am, I didn't need to take the MMPI to tell me that."

She remained wholly unimpressed with my stab at humor and continued, "Secondly," she said, "you have an anxiety disorder and attendant depression."

A new fear suddenly shot through me like a bullet and shattered the uneasy peace I had made with myself during the previous year. I had taught myself to believe that I had been cured. I had even convinced myself that such "non-sense" was the truth. Ten thirty-minute sessions and a half a bottle of Valium was all that I needed. I was certain of that. In fact, had not my first psychiatrist himself noted that I was doing better? I did not want to hear more, but this professional was far from finished with her report. Her words were to bring even more pain.

"Sir, you are not nearly as smart as you think you are." Here I mounted a wholly ineffectual defense by mumbling something like, "Then I must really be stupid in that I've never considered myself to be much smarter than a ground hog sticking his head out of some burrow to determine which way the wind is blowing. "

She arose in stately silence, extended her hand in mock reverence, and as I her took her hand into my trembling fingers, she offered one biting word of backhanded comfort. She said in a voice only slightly above a whisper, "You might consider selling insurance. I think you could be very good at it."

I was devastated. There was a part of me that fully expected her to congratulate me on my innate brilliance and then compliment me on my new found psychological integration, or "togetherness." As I stumbled out of the woman's office, I felt a close to inconsolable pain sweep through my entire being.

I desperately wanted to be accepted, yet I was not wise or honest enough to realize that acceptance has nothing whatsoever to do with perfection. It never has and it never will. But to me, perfection was the single "savior," if you will, potent enough in my unhealthy way of thinking to deliver me to the threshold of the acceptance I so desperately craved. And what I longed for most, and could not figure out how to manufacture, no matter how hard I tried, was some semblance of inner peace.

I was broken. This woman had peered deep into my wounds and in her rather austere manner shared with me what her tests and inventories declared to her to be my truth.

I longed to be perfect. More, I was convinced that I needed to be perfect. The harder I tried, the more terror I engendered. All that I could figure out to do was to turn up the volume on my efforts. Consequently, I sought perfection even more diligently while I battled with my natural

Step 1: I am powerless.

laziness, depression, and fear. It was a miserable existence.

Help was at my fingertips, but I failed to discover it. Answers lay in the Scripture, but I did not know that. I was far too consumed with learning the original languages of the Bible and with sounding impressive to pause long enough to discover the truth in the ancient texts that were waiting to shepherd me toward healing.

A few years ago, psychiatrist M. Scott Peck authored a book entitled *A World Waiting to Be Born.* I so wish that I had had access to this man's thinking during my seminary days, but in truth, even had he been pumping out life-affecting books and tapes back then, I suspect that I would have paid little attention. No, back then, I was far too obsessed with the god of perfectionism to heed his, as well as the Scripture's, call to grace. Here I was preparing for the Gospel ministry, where grace is not only the natural climate of the kingdom I was preparing myself to proclaim, but also the best news this world could ever receive.

In *A World Waiting to Be Born,* Scott Peck employs a powerful reference from the Old Testament (2 Sam. 9) to describe the human condition. Peck writes:

> *After Saul and Jonathan were slain by the Philistines, what little remained of the House of Saul went into hiding and David was made king over Israel. A few years pass before David learns that Jonathan had a son, Mephibosheth, a crippled youth, surviving in squalor in an outcast camp. Because of his covenant with Jonathan, David has the young cripple brought to him, and not only restores his land but invites the lad to always dine with him amid the splendor of the king's table. Mephibosheth apparently does so, but then shortly vanishes to return to the outcast camp. Many more years pass, and suddenly one day Mephibosheth, in rags, shows up once again at King David's palace. When David asks him why he left, Mephibosheth in essence replies, 'My people told me you were not to be trusted, and I believed them. I thought it was too good to be true. But after watching you from afar I have come to realize, even though I do not deserve it, that your charity, your love and covenant, is for real.' And so it was that the poor, lame man returned to the splendor of the royal table.*[1]

So what is the point? To me it is this: we are all Mephibosheths. We have all been invited to dine daily at the royal table, but we have no more notion of that invitation than a pig has an appreciation for German opera. We are woefully ignorant of the fact that we are invited to any kind of table other than the one at which we park our misery on a daily basis.

Like Mephibosheth, we are all crippled in one way or another. None of us are perfect. Not one of us! We are so full of pride that we remain wholly unwilling to trust the divine invitation that has been issued to us, just as King David long ago issued a kingly invitation to another crippled man. Throughout our lives we ignore and, thereby, decline the invitation; thus we remove ourselves from the royal table and remain lonely and, in the deepest part of our being, terrified.

Just as the message of a covenant came to Jonathan's son in the form of an invitation, the message of grace comes to us in a similar form. Like the crippled Mephibosheth, we are free to trust God and we are also free to doubt that this invisible, mysterious force we call God is to be trusted. The choice is entirely ours. If we are willing to trust, we may then dine at the royal table. If we respond to the invitation with a polite "No, thank you," we can scramble about seeking security on our own terms and trusting only ourselves. Again, the choice is totally ours.

One other powerful insight into the nature of humanity is found in chapter 32 of the Book of Genesis, verse 24. My own experience resonates to this ancient legend in that it feels to me that I, like Jacob, the protagonist in this tale, have invested a good bit of my life wrestling with some kind of angel.

And Jacob was left alone; and a man wrestled with him until the breaking of the day. When the man saw that he did not prevail against Jacob, he touched the hollow of his thigh; and Jacob's thigh was out of joint as he wrestled with him. Then he said, "Let me go for this day is breaking." But Jacob said, " I will not let you go, unless you bless me." And he said to him, "What is your name?" And he said, "Jacob." Then he said, "Your name shall no longer be called Jacob, but Israel, for you have striven with God and with men, and have prevailed." Then Jacob asked him, "Tell me, I pray, your name."
"Why is it that you ask my name?" And there he blessed him.[2]

What should we make of this bizarre story? To me, it is similar to the tale I paraphrased from 2 Samuel in that, like Mephibosheth, Jacob is crippled. What is the point of this comparison? It is this. To be a human being means to be crippled, which I interpret as a biblical euphemism for "being imperfect." Yes, Jacob did prevail, but he was crippled by the struggle.

The ancient wisdom in these stories communicates clearly that perfectionism, and our striving for it, is nothing more than a cultural myth with no roots in reality. We are crippled, all of us. Imperfection is our very nature, and it is this state, if you will, that places us in dire need of the greatest gift we could receive—grace. If we were not crippled, we would have no need for God or for God's healing gift of grace.

Step 1: I am powerless.

Mephibosheth ran and hid, and Jacob wrestled with an angel until daybreak. I am convinced that most of us, like Mephibosheth, do not trust readily, and like Jacob, we, because we lack trust, spend our days striving with God in the darkness.

Another fascinating facet of the Jacob story is the reference to the struggle's lasting until dawn. For me, this is the ancient mytho-poetic, and very powerful, symbol of the shift in our human struggle from unconsciousness to consciousness. I further submit that it was no accident that the man (or the angel) in this story felt no obvious motivation to terminate his wrestling match with Jacob until the break of day. And keep in mind that it was at the break of day in this old Hebrew tale that the blessing was finally received.

The same, I believe, is true for us. We struggle with our own unconsciousness, which in my view is precisely what the writer of Genesis is declaring here. Our struggle with the unconscious is synonymous to our struggle with God. And when the day finally breaks, when consciousness finally dawns, it is then, and only then, that we receive a blessing.

And what is that blessing? Essentially, it is that we come to recognize two truths. First, we discover who we truly are. That is, we come to know our own name. And it is through that painful, wounding discovery that we come to understand that a big part of our identity is our "crippled" condition.

In short, what I believe Scripture is teaching us in these stories is that it is only through a striving with God that we come to know that, like it or not, we must trust God completely. Our imperfect condition absolutely requires it. We must depend entirely upon grace. That is our true condition.

But the rub is this. I do not want to trust. I have learned the hard way not to trust. I have trusted colleagues who have turned against me and tried to besmirch a reputation that I probably cherish far too much. I have trusted friends to maintain confidentiality, and they have disappointed me by sharing liberally those details that I held to be sacred between us. I have trusted professors and supervisors to be rigorous in their critique of my work, and they have disappointed me by offering formulas in place of insight. Once, when I was a kid, I even trusted a docile old bull, which quite by coincidence was also named Jacob, not to chase me as I crossed his domain on my way to a fishing hole. Quite out of character, he did, in fact, chase me.

No, I do not want to trust, but both the Mephibosheth and the Jacob stories suggest to me, at least, that trust is the essential ingredient in any realistic experience with grace. But I do not want to admit to myself, to God, and certainly not to another human being that I must trust God. No, I would much rather live with the illusion that I am not a cripple, and the truth is, I would rather wrestle a skunk than admit to my own imperfections.

After all, I pay my bills on time. My credit rating is sterling. The IRS has never been on my back. I have been judged a success at most every job I've ever held. Heck, the mayor of Dallas once declared before the city council that I had made as much of an impact on the city as any single minister in that community's history. Therefore, I do not find it at all attractive, appealing, or even necessary, for that matter, to admit that some part of my life does not work, or that I must trust God because I am by nature imperfect.

I have spent my whole life being powerful. Such a position was, it seems, the perceived assignment, if not the destiny, of every red-blooded American male raised in the postwar cultural milieu that served as the context for my ascendancy to the throne of narcissism. Therefore, I adamantly refuse to admit my powerlessness over almost everything. In employing the biblical imagery of both 2 Samuel and Genesis, I find it distasteful to embrace, even as a remote possibility, any serious thought that I might somehow be crippled, or blemished, or less than perfect, and, therefore, in need of grace.

The truth is, of course, that I am very crippled, and like Mephibosheth, I, too, have been invited to a royal table. The only problem is that to sit down at that table, I must first trust. Like Jacob, I, too, have invested a dark night in struggling, wrestling, and striving with God. When the dawn finally broke in my own unconscious warfare, I was compelled to admit that, like my spiritual ancestors Jacob and Mephibosheth, I, too, am wounded. Therefore, like those before and around me, I stand in constant need of something or someone much greater than I.

This is the recognition that brings us to the first Step of our healing. We must admit that we are crippled. We must also embrace the truth that we cannot make our lives work through sheer will power because we are powerless over so much. Some of us are powerless over alcohol. Others are powerless over an addiction to control, fear, sex, relationships, what we perceive to be love, and countless other objects of attachment.

But the fundamental truth is that we are powerless, and the deeper, even more ominous, truth is that our healing is predicated *entirely* upon our willingness to recognize our broken nature and then to trust God. I can trust that the invitation to dine at the royal table is genuine, or I can ignore it for a lifetime and hide, like Mephibosheth.

Step 1: I am powerless.

I have heard it said that all truth is discovered (this idea will be discussed more fully in later chapters). I suspect that notion is correct. In my view, truth cannot be taught; it must be discovered. I firmly believe this. Therefore, I cannot possibly discover someone else's need for grace or that person's path to the royal table. No, this path toward healing is invariably an excruciatingly difficult and personal striving. Each person must come to grips with his or her own truth, his or her personal need for grace.

Having offered that perspectival preface, to use a ten-dollar word I learned in seminary, I would, however, invite you to take some time to write down how it is that your life has become unmanageable. This list indicates your willingness, caused by your striving with God, to make notes regarding your crippled condition.

I believe that, as you become increasingly honest with yourself and, like Jacob, as you strive with God in the darkness of your unconsciousness, you will discover your own reality. Wherever you find that your life has become unmanageable, pause and dig down, as if you were digging for a spring beneath a stand of cottonwoods in a desert. With time, patience, and courage, you may discover what it is that you are powerless over. At that point, you will experience a dawn similar to the one that long ago broke over Jacob's struggle with the angel. The blessings, though, are the same for you and for me as they were for Jacob.

If you keep after it, you, like Jacob, will no doubt learn the truth. And through this tussle, as we called a struggle in East Texas, you will likely discover the truth of your own identity. In the words of Genesis, you will come to know your very name. This knowledge is a great yet painful blessing that remains mysteriously, but inextricably, connected to our suffering.

While digging, it is helpful, I believe, to pay careful attention to the words of the spiritual giants who have preceded us. Listen to the Apostle Paul as he writes to the Church at Rome (and to us) as it is recorded in Romans, seventh chapter, verses 14–20 RSV:

> *We know that the law is spiritual; but I am carnal, sold under sin. I do not understand my own actions. For I do not do what I want, but I do the very thing that I hate. Now if I do what I do not want, I agree that the law is good. So it is then no longer I that do it, but sin which dwells within me. For I know that nothing good dwells within me, that is, in my flesh. I can will what is right, but I cannot do it. For I do not do the good I want, but the evil I do not want is what I do. Now if I do what I do not want, it is no longer I that do it, but sin which dwells within me.*

He continues in verse 24: "Wretched man that I am! Who will deliver me from this body of death? Thanks be to God through Jesus Christ our Lord! So then, I of myself serve the law of God with my mind, but with my flesh I serve the law of sin."

When Paul writes that he can will what is right but cannot do it, I long to jump to my feet and raise a loud amen. What I believe the apostle is writing about is what those of us who are working recovery discover in Step 1. This might be something of a stretch, but I submit that his sentiment is about as close to Step 1 as a leaner is to a ringer in horseshoes.

In a very real sense Paul is proclaiming to his fellow Christians in Rome that he is powerless to do what is right. Of course, his words are far more eloquent than most of us will ever write, but I agree fully with his assessment of his overall condition. It is my condition as well. If I have learned anything in my long-night's striving in the darkness of my unconsciousness, it is this: in those areas of my life where I am powerless, I cannot always will myself to do what needs to be done. I have tried, and I have come up empty most every time.

As I mentioned earlier, and as I will write again, I cannot will myself out of my fear addiction. Believe me, I have given it my best shot. Nothing has worked. The more I have struggled to overcome it, the more exhausted, resentful, and frightened I have become. No, I am very like Mephibosheth, Jacob, and the apostle Paul. I am a cripple struggling in the darkness to learn my identity and to gain control of my life in the important context of doing what is healthy. Like the apostle, I have discovered that in many areas I am not in control. What's more, part of my life is now, and has been for years, quite out of control.

For years, I have been grateful to the apostle Paul for his steadfast faith. Since discovering recovery, I have grown to appreciate even more this man's courage. Employing the language of this century, I have come to view what he accomplished in this poignant letter as nothing less than taking his 1st Step before the congregation of the Church at Rome.

I am equally satisfied that for the rest of my life I will remain grateful for this man's willingness to be bold in his proclamation of what was, for him, his own discovered truth following a striving with God through the dark night.

Some years ago, I attended a lecture at the Presbyterian Seminary on a February evening when sleet and slick streets were prophesied. Of course, I did not expect many folks to be present in that the weather was threatening to turn in the direction of somewhere between inhospitable and dangerous.

As I entered the tiny seminary chapel, I was amazed to discover it

Step 1: I am powerless.

packed. I wondered about the wisdom of staying. Since I began this discipline of recovery, however, I have chosen to listen to internal stirrings that seem to direct me regularly to this sort of meeting. Something deep within me whispered, not in words so much as with bumps and nudges, that I should be in that chapel to hear whoever was scheduled to speak on this cold night.

A minister who was touted as a gifted storyteller rather than a noted academician ascended into the pulpit, cleared his throat, gazed down upon his expectant audience, and said something like this: "The problem is this: God is desperately seeking us and we are desperately seeking to be God."

In that moment I recognized why I was supposed to be in that man's presence. In that one sentence he offered me what the author of Genesis described: our striving with God in the dark of the night.

For the whole of my life, I have attempted to get my emotional needs met. So have you. Such is the nature of us human beings. When I perceived that many of these needs would not be met, I became frightened in some subterranean part of my being. My unconscious pattern then became to turn up the volume on my efforts. The result was, of course, that I worked to exert even more power in the effort of getting these needs met. In the process, I became more cunning, manipulative, coercive, and controlling of my immediate environment.

Unconsciously, I learned in the process to equate my ego with power. Quite unwittingly, I also learned, and later embraced, a very dangerous heresy. I taught myself to believe in myself as power. Therefore, at a very early age, I further grounded my ego in the dangerous illusion that I might exert control over *every* area of my life.

The process of learning inevitably breeds the illusion of personal control over life in most of us, and we cling tighter than the jaws on a snapping turtle to that illusion. Out of one side of our mouth we profess an insincere, pious, and amorphous assent to some kind of a god, but the truth is that all along the way of our development we are more comfortable confessing our strong allegiance to the conviction that life works best for us when we trust *only* in ourselves.

It was to this very dilemma, I believe, that the man in the seminary chapel spoke to me so eloquently on that icy February evening. What he offered me was both good and terrifying news. The good news is, of course, that even though I have made a mess of this sacred gift called life, there is still one out there who also dwells in the core of my own broken heart, one who always seeks me.

The problem with this good news is that it brings me back to the issue of trust. In order for me to permit myself to be sought, I must give up—"surrender" is the word we employ in the 12 Steps—the very notion that I am most tempted to believe, namely, that I am powerful and, therefore, can control my life.

In the years I have actively practiced the principles of the 12 Steps, I have come to believe that I can control only about 5 percent of my life. That is roughly the part of my existence that seems to lie within the limits of what psychology terms my "ego boundaries." This 5 percent includes, among other issues, my thoughts, my feelings, my behavior, the quality of my relationship with God, and my right treatment of neighbors. The rest of my life, I have come to believe, belongs wholly to God.

So the man in the seminary pulpit was as right as two rabbits, as an old black East Texas sharecropper taught me to say before I was old enough to read. God is always chasing after us. All that we have to do is get out of the "God business" and let God be God.

It all sounds simple enough. But as I heard folks in the Piney Woods of East Texas say when I was a boy, it sure ain't easy. To get out of the God business means that I must let go and once again surrender the illusion of my own power. Simply put, I must unlearn what I have invested a lifetime in learning, what I have embraced and defended as my "truth."

This 1st Step is anything but easy. It is simple, but it is also scary, maddening, frustrating, and more slippery than new ice on a winter sidewalk. My greatest fear about this Step is that if I practice it with any sense of integrity, I will still not get my emotional needs met. The incontrovertible truth is, however, that by doing life *my* way, I have *never* gotten those needs met in any healthy way, and I have certainly not made my life work.

Doing it *my* way, though, is all that I know to do. It is not easy to learn a whole new, even paradoxical, way of thinking, but that is precisely what the 1st Step requires—a radical (meaning rooted) new orientation to what it means to live this life. Step 1, then, in my mind, is the beginning Step of nothing less than a spiritual conversion from an ego-centered faith to a soul-centered life. Step 1 is standing before God, a mirror, and before other human beings and saying exactly what that gifted storyteller offered from that hand-carved seminary pulpit. It is to admit that I have not permitted God to catch me because I have been far too busy at playing God to permit myself such intimacy with the Truth.

I do not know of many confessions that are more frightening than the one required in Step 1. And I do not know of any perspective that can bring more healing and more inner peace than to admit that I can no longer be my own God.

Step 1: I am powerless.

Some years ago I directed a soup kitchen in the bowels of a Presbyterian church in downtown Dallas. The purpose of this ministry was to offer food, clothing, and compassion to the hundreds, at times, thousands of men, women, and children who subsisted on the streets of that prosperous city.

Over the years it became my practice to listen almost daily to the broken hearts and disordered souls of those men and women who were struggling with the disease of alcoholism. Once again, permit me to reiterate that during the course of my decade of service to the poor and to those whom Jesus once described as "the least of these," it never once dawned on me that I shared their disease. In truth, and in retrospect, I now understand that our symptoms were markedly different, but the disease was the same.

One particular morning hangs in my memory like a kite in a billowy March sky. I am not certain why I remember this episode so vividly because I enjoyed commerce with literally thousands of desperate folks in those ten years, but I recall the details of this event as though it were yesterday.

A man named Earl approached me at the soup kitchen and through his watery, rum-soaked gaze, I sensed more pain in his soul than any man should ever cause himself to endure. He staggered before me. For several awkward moments he said nothing. He dropped his eyes to the floor, shuffled, waited, and then said, "Pastor, I'm dying out here on these streets. Please help me."

"What do you want me to do?" I asked.

"Get me into the Sally's [Salvation Army's] detox program."

My standard response to such requests was summed up to Earl in these words: "Okay, Earl, you come back here tomorrow and present yourself to me in a sober condition, and I'll find you a detox program, I promise."

Twenty-four hours later he appeared at my office door as sober as a barn owl. I smiled at him in silent appreciation of the effort he had made to begin his own healing. I then pointed to the parking lot and said, "Let's go, Earl."

We drove in near silence toward what was then the downtown location of the Salvation Army. When we arrived, he and I climbed out of my Toyota, and I watched with interest as he shambled down the sidewalk in obvious determination to seek healing from what he now regarded as a terminal disease.

As he placed his hand on the large, wooden door knob, he turned to me and with enough sadness written across his face to devastate even the heartiest human heart, he whispered, "I can't."

With those two words, he let go of the door, reached deep inside his overcoat, and extracted a full jug of some cheap poison he had obviously purchased prior to his arrival on my doorstep. I watched with a mixture of anger and sadness as he twisted the plastic lid and lifted the bottle to his lips. In no more than a half dozen chugs, the contents of that ugly jug disappeared.

He staggered, wiped the residue of the cheap wine from his grizzled face, and offered his apology one last time. "I can't, Pastor. I just can't!"

Countless times in my own dark night of the soul I have heard Earl's words ringing in my ears and resonating with my unwillingness to trust enough to live life in a way that admits that I can no longer be God.

Please hear no judgment in my tale of Earl. He and I share the identical disease. If there is a difference between us, in addition to the manifestation of our symptoms, it is that I have been blessed with people in my life who have comforted and forgiven me as well as confronted me with the truth of my own disease. I seriously doubt, though I have no way of knowing for certain, that Earl could have made any similar claim for such support.

In my conscious awareness, I never judged him. I simply stood there alone on that Dallas sidewalk and recognized a truth that I would embrace as my own in the years to come: the 1st Step is not easy. It is simple, but it is not easy. Obviously, Earl was not willing to make that initial step toward recovery, and for close to another decade, neither was I.

In many ways it is not helpful to employ what I have come to term "the Earl episode" as a valid illustration of the difficulty we face in taking the 1st Step and in recognizing our powerlessness over our need to be God. The vast majority of the folks I know, and the population who will likely read this book, have not slipped into the gutter that Earl knew on a daily basis. Unlike Earl, the readers of this book do not live on skid row. They are not dependent upon a soup kitchen for their daily bread, and most who will read this book do not stand in dire need of some detoxification program.

Therefore, the Earl episode fails to make much impression upon our self-awareness. To us, it is quite understandable that a wino or street bum, as Earl was termed, might be an alcoholic. In fact, his appearance provides us with the ammunition for all manner of denial. We can gaze upon the Earls of this world and convince ourselves rather easily that we are healthy while it is the poor devils of this world, such as Earl, who are devoured by this disease we know as alcoholism. When we hear of the likes of Earl, our pride immediately tends to take over, and suddenly we self-righteously perceive of ourselves as *very* different from the likes of Earl.

Trappist monk Thomas Merton warns us against such pride in these profound words: "In every man [and woman] there is hidden some root of despair because in every man [or woman] there is a pride that vegetates and springs weeds and rank flowers of self-pity as soon as our own resources fail us. But because our own resources inevitably fail us, we are all more or less subject to discouragement and to despair."[3]

Thomas Merton is right. Our own resources invariably fail us whether we are successful, competent business people or shuffling about in a state of perpetual inebriation like my friend Earl.

Our resources inevitably fail us.

Permit me to share yet another story, one that will hit much closer to home, I suspect. A few days prior to my taking a writing retreat in the Texas Hill Country, I received a phone call from a middle-aged woman requesting that I see her, her son, and her husband for a counseling session. In my most polished pastoral tone, I informed the woman that I was no longer taking new clients. I did, however, agree to meet with them once as a family so that I might make some kind of assessment of their need and then refer them to one of several therapists I have come to respect here in Austin. It was interesting to me that this woman informed me that her husband was willing to come to my office because he had heard me speak. I correctly, it turns out, read her comment to mean that he did not respect many folks in the helping professions.

As the couple entered my office, I noticed that the sharp lines in the man's face formed what appeared to me to be angular features suggesting a long history of anger, or perhaps even rage. I sensed in this man a driving energy that he held in check under only the thinnest veneer of civility.

The woman offered as her complaint her view that there was far too much tension in the home. Her husband's view was, of course, quite different. He was not at all concerned about the tension. No. What bothered him to the point of near apoplexy was that his honor student son had chosen to enroll in what I suppose might be most accurately described as a small, mediocre college in New England. This man was incredulous at his son's decision. As he sat before me, I watched the blush rising to his face, suggesting a deepening awareness of the obvious discomfort he was, no doubt, experiencing. I broke a brief and queasy silence with this question: "Is the school accredited?"

"Yes," the father admitted in a tone that sounded surprisingly subdued.

"Well, then, what is the problem?" I asked. "It's not like he is signing up to join the Klan or some bizarre religious cult."

The father stunned me by pounding his knee with his fist, and in a voice boiling with rage, he exclaimed, "But it is not the best. And this boy of mine needs to be doing the best."

I never know much about what is really happening within human beings. The best any of us can do is offer an educated guess. My guess is that this father is suffering from the identical disease that has Earl and that long ago claimed my own soul. He presented me his anger, but I suspect that deep down he is a terrified little boy who has never, at least not for very long, probed his own unconscious to discover the source of this nearly unbearable pain. Like me, he is a Mephibosheth hiding from the royal table, and he is also a Jacob striving with God in the darkness. All that he seems to be aware of is that his gifted son is "not doing his best!"

In a very real sense, this man, like most of us, is walking around unconscious. Oh, he rises in the morning, slips into his trousers, buttons his shirt, and knots a necktie, but this man is in many ways as unconscious as he was when he lay in bed next to his sleeping wife an hour before he awakened to the ordinary morning routine. In my view, this man is gripped by fear. His defense, most likely, is the same as mine: to seek to be God. In fact, my own read on this man, which again is purely subjective and therefore prone to error, is that he is every bit as sick as either my friend from the street, Earl, or me.

There is one important difference, though. Earl, through the trauma brought about by his symptoms, had become conscious. He was not willing to confess his powerlessness over alcohol, but he was aware of the disease when he came to me seeking help. The man in my office, on the other hand, remains wholly unconscious of the issue of his fear. He is walking around, but still, from my own perspective and in my own judgment, he remains unconscious regarding that force that has captured his soul.

Scott Peck speaks of this condition of becoming conscious. "When we ate the apple of the Tree of Knowledge of Good and Evil, we became conscious, and having become conscious, we immediately became self-conscious."[4]

Consciousness is the solitary path out of the disease and into the initial Step. It is ironic to me that Earl was conscious and that the man who came to me to complain about his son's enrollment in a perfectly adequate college was unconscious. Earl is, in the perception of our society, nothing more than a skid row bum eking out an existence in what I now

Step 1: I am powerless.

believe is an existential purgatory, but still Earl remains conscious. His problem was that he was simply not ready to take Step 1. As he stood at the door of the Salvation Army, he recognized that he was not willing to admit that he was powerless over anything and that his life had become unmanageable.

On the other hand, the angry (actually, frightened) man who came to my office with his wife and adolescent son is by every measure of the cultural yardstick a roaring success. He owns his home, he makes his car payments on time, each year he satisfies Caesar's voracious appetite for taxes, and, in my presence, he professed to being an active and, by his own report, tithing layman in his church. But in my view, the man remained as unconscious as a sleeping baby. Unlike Adam, Eve, and my friend from the streets, this angry, profoundly frightened man had yet to taste of the tree of knowledge of good and evil.

Earl knew he needed help, but he was not willing to make that first necessary, terrifying step required for healing. The father in my office no more knew that he needed any kind of help than a turkey knows in October that Thanksgiving is not far off.

If we are to move toward healing, we must first become conscious. Consciousness is the necessary preface to Step 1. I must realize that I am in pain, perhaps even prodigious pain, and I must embrace the fact that some portion of my life is woefully out of control. It is only then, with such recognition under my belt, that I dare to ask for the only help that can possibly save me and deliver me to sanity.

A story from my childhood illustrates what it means to become conscious of the need of asking for help. One summer afternoon, my brother Bill and I were assigned by our mother to walk through the bucolic postwar neighborhood of Elmwood, in South Dallas, until we arrived at Mr. Dodd's barbershop. Bill was eight, and I was five. In Mom's estimation, we both stood in dire need of a haircut. By Bill's edict, I climbed up into Mr. Dodd's barber chair first and within minutes I was armed with a fresh, close-cropped haircut.

Because I have always been driven by what has been described as an uncommon curiosity, I decided to abandon the safety of the barbershop as Bill was treated to fifteen minutes of Mr. Dodd's professional attention. I wandered outside, just beyond the front door and behind an evaporative cooler that pumped cool, as opposed to cold, air into the barbershop.

For reasons that remain locked in my unconscious, I decided to stick my hand down a pipe that was firmly rooted in the sidewalk. Immediately I realized that I had made a terrible mistake. The pipe grabbed my arm and refused to let go. At first I tugged and squirmed, working to extricate my right arm from the vise grip of that vicious pipe. The harder I pulled, the tighter the pipe seemed to squeeze.

Soon enough, an entire barbershop full of customers, along with three barbers, including Mr. Dodd, had spilled out onto the sidewalk and were busily plotting and scheming as to how they might extricate my arm from the pipe. Unbeknownst to me, Bill was sprinting home, where he breathlessly, no doubt, informed our mother as to the details of my dilemma. While he was gone, a fat man wearing an undershirt and fancy suspenders which were holding up his sizable pleated slacks bent over the locus of my misery and said something like, "I know one little boy who just might lose his arm."

The man had no sooner finished terrorizing me than my father appeared on the sidewalk. He smiled as he walked toward me. He grabbed my arm just below the elbow and without a word of warning, he yanked. I remember him saying something about not sticking my arm in the sidewalk pipe again as he disappeared from view so that he might make a hasty return to his office downtown.

I never did stick my arm into that sidewalk pipe again, but I sure have in the past nearly half century gotten myself stuck in all manner of messes, most of which have been symptomatic of the disease of alcoholism. And only because I have come to believe that God's grace is as real as my father's grip upon my small arm have I been liberated.

This is Step 1. We must become conscious of the fact that our symptoms teach us a great, wonderful, and, at the same time, very painful lesson. We must also come to recognize that we cannot possibly extricate ourselves from the pipes into which we have foolishly shoved our arms. There is one, though, who is more than willing to yank us out of that rusty pipe. The requirement for liberation is simple: we must first be willing to ask. And therein lies the problem, because our pride slips in and distracts us from the honesty that healing invariably requires.

Step 1 is this: I must admit that I am, by nature, crippled. Therefore, I must also admit that I am not God, but that I stand in constant need of God's grace. Further, I must confess that I am powerless over whatever has me in its grip. Finally, I must recognize the truth that a part, if not all, of my life has become unmanageable.

It is quite simple to assent to those words, but it is never easy to take this difficult, wonderful Step. May God grant all of us the courage to keep taking this Step in full knowledge that perfection, especially in the context of recovery, is nothing more than a myth.

Step 1 is the place where we begin our slow process of healing. I im-

Step 1: I am powerless.

plore you to admit your powerlessness over whatever it is that brings you misery. In this crucial admission, be gentle with yourself, be patient, and, above all, trust in the truth that God is *always* on the side of your healing.

References

[1] M. Scott Peck, *A World Waiting to Be Born* (New York: Bantam Books, 1993), p. 57.

[2] Genesis 32:24-29 RSV.

[3] Thomas Merton, *New Seeds of Contemplation* (New York: New Directions Books, 1961), p. 180.

[4] M. Scott Peck, *Further Along the Road Less Traveled* (New York: Simon and Shuster, 1993), p. 18.

2

I love thee, Oh Lord, my strength. The Lord is my rock, and my fortress, and my deliverer, my God, my rock, in whom I take refuge, my shield, and the horn of my salvation, my stronghold. I call upon the Lord, who is worthy to be praised.

Psalm 18:1–3 RSV

Step 2:   I believe that a power (I say God as revealed in Jesus Christ) greater than me can restore me to sanity.

Recently, I happened upon the startling statistic that we Americans compose 4 percent of the world's population, yet we consume 64 percent of the illicit drugs in this world.[1] When I finished reading that unsettling fact, I fell back into my office chair, rubbed my eyes with my shirt sleeve in the cause of making certain that they were focusing clearly, and then posed one of those useless, unanswerable questions to which I alluded in the introduction. Why? I bellowed louder than a hungry calf separated by a barbed wire fence from its mother. Why?

Of course, my response is that I do not own the reasons underlying such stunning data. I simply don't know. But I do believe that we, the people of this nation, are experiencing a revolution the magnitude of which has never been seen or felt by any population.

I suspect that there are as many theories as to the genesis of our obvious predilection for and fascination with illicit drugs as there are folks available and trained to hammer out those ideas on the anvils of responsible research. I simply don't possess even one plausible theory. But I do sense that who we are today could accurately be described as a society tottering on the very precipice of insanity.

Simply put, the statistic tells me that we have become one insane culture. Of course, not every one of us is insane, but if we believe the above statistic, there are a bunch of us who, consciously or unconsciously, hold to the truth that our individual salvation is to be found in a pill, an injection, or a bottle.

That conviction is as old as the mythical Garden, but today it is being financed by a prosperous people who, unfortunately, just may possess more dollars than sense. Because of historical determinants that have placed this nation's economy at center stage in the global political arena, we have positioned ourselves to purchase all manner of high-powered manufactured gods. These deities serve us well *temporarily* in that they are quite capable of relieving boredom, bolstering confidence, and eliminating depression, but in time their effects wear off and they leave us with nothing more than a deeper craving for some kind of peace.

In effect, what we do when we worship at the throne of chemical dependency, or of any kind of dependency, for that matter, is to align ourselves with death. We may call it salvation, but in fact it is something very different. We may worship with our energy, our time, our passion, and, of course, our money, but dependency of any kind can never liberate us. It will serve only to strangle and eventually to suffocate us until we finally succumb to death.

Initially, we die spiritually when we worship at the throne of the god of chemical dependency. We fail to love, and then we lose sight of what it means to love altogether. In time, addiction destroys our bodies as well as our spirit and our minds, and ultimately we die a physical death long after we have experienced the demise of our spirit. Until the very end, the disease tricks us into believing that we are living, when in truth the existence we experience is a painful, torturous death.

In the recovery program we say that the disease is known by three descriptors, or adjectives: (1) cunning, (2) powerful, and (3) pervasive. The trick that addiction plays on us in convincing us that death is life, in my perspective, is prima facie evidence of precisely what it means when we say that the disease is cunning. And because the disease is cunning, powerful, and pervasive, it possesses the power to make us insane. Make no mistake about that.

I find the words in Step 2 to be the most comforting words in all 12 Steps. For years I desperately needed to know that something or some-

Step 2: God can restore me to sanity.

one could return me to sanity. Even more, I suppose, I longed to know that sanity, for me, was even a possibility.

In that I am a Christian, I have made Jesus Christ my own model for what it means to be sane. Now let me be clear here and state that the Christ who is the model for my sanity is not what I term the "cultural Christ" of the dollar-and-holler televangelists who scare us with hellfire and then comfort us with threadbare platitudes and hollow promises of salvation on the far side of some river. No, the Christ of my model for sanity is the Christ of my own discovery as he is to be found in the scriptures.

Many who read this book have, I suspect, been abused by preachers or even by parents in the context of so-called Christian love. They have been so beat up with a Jesus who never existed except in the imagination of some angry parent, repressed Sunday school teacher, or perverse preacher that the very mention of the name Jesus sends chills crawling up their spines.

I was not abused in that way, but I have worked with scores of folks who were. Therefore, I say to you before you decide to toss this chapter in the air and run for your favorite palliative behavior, *please* do yourself the favor of discovering the Christ in the New Testament. Make it a part of your daily discipline to read a section of one of the four Gospel narratives until you have completed one entire book. (Mark is only sixteen brief chapters.)

My hunch is that you will discover in Jesus Christ a man who was very human, therefore credible, and, most of all, sane. Jesus gave us the greatest commandment for sanity that, in my view, has ever been offered to humanity. It admonishes us to love God with every bit of energy we can muster and to love our neighbors as we love ourselves.

My grandfather, who was a sage, and in the estimation of the whole of my family, probably the sanest man any of us ever knew, once offered me this proverb in the milking pen: "Bobby," he said, "don't ever try to sit on a two-legged stool."

I must have been no older than eight at the time, but I held onto those words and pondered them often until I arrived at seminary, where I was privileged to study the New Testament in its original language, Koine Greek. And one summer afternoon, more than a decade and a half following my grandfather's gift to me of that mysterious proverb, I was reading the New Testament in the seminary library when I happened upon what we have come to know as the "Great Commandment." Once again, Jesus was exalting me, this time in Greek, to love God and to love my neighbor as I love myself. For me the riddle I had learned in Granddaddy's milking pen was finally solved. This Great Commandment of Jesus Christ, I decided on the third floor of the Stitt Library at Austin Presbyterian Theological Library, was precisely what Granddaddy meant by a three-legged stool.

If we give more attention to loving God than we give to loving ourselves or our neighbors, we will tumble off of the two-legged stool and fall into the muck of the cow pen. If we love ourselves too much, which is known in clinical circles as narcissism, and we fail to give attention to loving God, we also quickly tumble off of the stool. If we love our neighbors and not ourselves and God with equal measure, we will once again fall. I figure this last configuration is what is known in cultural/clinical circles as "codependency."

No, to be sane, we must sit squarely on a three-legged stool supported by the love of God, the love of neighbor, and the love of ourselves.

For years the three-legged stool has proven a most helpful image for me. There is only one problem with it. You see, to be perfectly honest, I have a real problem in loving God because I have a greater problem trusting God. If I am to proclaim that I love God, then I must also be willing to back that claim up with the willingness to trust the one I profess to love. That, in my mind, is the fundamental difference between Jesus and me. Jesus trusted God completely; I don't.

Until very recently I did not understand that I was an idolater. The truth is that I am. I attended seminary and was even ordained into the Presbyterian Church up in the Arkansas Ozarks, but for the whole of my life I have been an idolater. I have given lip service to trusting God and for close to a quarter of a century I have proclaimed the "good news" of Jesus Christ to others. But through it all, I have, in fact, worshiped regularly at the throne of any god whom I believed could deliver me to any place where I might find even temporary relief from the fear that tore at my soul.

I have come to believe that what we worship is a personal god. A partial list of my current gods is as follows: prestige, fame, acceptance, affirmation, harmony (or lack of interpersonal conflict), success symbols, respect, and, most of all, financial security.

I have heard it said by not a few people in a variety of ways that Jesus was not really tempted in that, in truth, he was really God. The implication underlying this kind of thinking, of course, is that Jesus was merely "playing" at being human. Nothing could be farther from the truth. This particular heresy is but one of the reasons I encourage you to return to the Gospel narratives to discover the authentic Christ of the Scripture.

I believe that if you will discipline yourself to make that discovery, you

Step 2: God can restore me to sanity.

will find a man who struggled with being obedient every bit as much as you and I are called upon to struggle with that same issue. Listen, if you will, to the passion contained in the 40th verse of Chapter 22 of Luke's Gospel, the story that precedes Jesus' arrest, mocking, humiliating trial, and execution at the hands of the Roman authorities: "And when he came to the place, he said to them, 'Pray that you may not enter into temptation.' And he withdrew from them about a stone's throw, and knelt down and prayed. 'Father if thou art willing, remove this cup from me; nevertheless, not my will, but thine be done'."

In popular parlance, it was in that garden that Jesus on his knees cashed a check that he had been writing for the previous three years. In truth, he did not want to do God's will in that painful moment in the garden. Who would? But he trusted God enough to grab hold of his faith as the single force powerful enough to penetrate his obvious terror. He chose obedience over a capitulation to fear, and a thoughtful, conscious response over an emotional reaction.

All too often we think of Jesus as some remote being who lived a pristine and perfect existence two millennia ago. In our imagination, we have removed him so far from our own experience that we truly believe that the standards he established are far beyond what we might live. "Why should I even try?" we ask ourselves. "After all, he was God and I am nothing more than a teacher, an attorney, a homemaker, a printer, a farmer, a bookkeeper. I cannot possibly live up to such impossible standards."

Jesus was a man. He was very human. The standards he established are the hallmarks of what it means to be a sane human being, but still he was fully a man. But make no mistake about it, while he was wholly a man, or a human being like you and me, he was also God. His godliness, however, did not remove him from the ubiquitous temptation to avoid pain.

Scott Peck describes well the personality and the humanity of Christ:

I discovered a man who was almost continually frustrated. His frustration leaps out of virtually every page. "What do I have to say to you? How many times do I have to say it? What do I have to do to get through to you?" I have also discovered a man who was frequently sad and sometimes depressed, frequently anxious and scared. A man who was prejudiced on one occasion, although He was able to overcome that prejudice and transcend it in healing love. A man who was terribly, terribly lonely, yet often desperately needed to be alone. I discovered a man so incredibly real that no one could have made Him up.[2]

Jesus struggled. Read these two words again, and I hope that you discover as much comfort in them as I do. Jesus struggled. I have struggled all of my adult life, but when I was no more than a shirttail kid jumping fresh-plowed furrows and being chased by old Jacob, our family bull, I must have convinced myself that adults had it together. I figured that when I became an adult, I would finally learn who I was and, most of all, who God was. In my mind back then, children and adolescents were exempted from such "divine" insight.

You can imagine my disappointment when I walked across the chancel in the chapel of a small liberal arts college and had conferred upon me a baccalaureate degree with the full, conscious recognition that I no more knew who I was and who God was than when I enrolled as a freshman. The pain of that disappointment was tolerable in that I was still young, full of energy, and free from the burdens of serious responsibility. Five years later, I walked across the chancel of another church to receive a second degree, this time, a divinity degree. My disappointment was even deeper. I hid the shame that welled inside my soul, but the truth was that, once again, I knew no more about myself, or about God, than when I began the three-year process known as theological education.

Months later, I was ordained in another chancel of the Presbyterian Church. This time I was close to panic in that the expectation now upon me was to articulate the truth of God's will from an informed position of at least minimal self-awareness. In truth, though I had graduated with honors from the seminary, I was not in a position to live up to this expectation.

I faked it for years and concealed my terror. In time I became a fairly popular speaker, but, in truth, every time I ventured forth somewhere to share the TRUTH with others, I would slink away from the experience even more convinced that I was a phony at best, and a liar at worst.

The ministry only exacerbated my terror. Counseling did me no real good in that I was never properly diagnosed. Finally, one day in the early stages of my recovery through working the 12 Steps one day at a time, it dawned on me that I am "in process." Sometime after that moment of revelation, I discovered that all of us are, in fact, *always* in process. Process is both part of our true nature and nothing less than a holy venture. Those among us who believe that they are not in process, in other words, who have convinced themselves that they are in possession of the "truth" are, in my mind, the most unhealthy, and perhaps even the most insane, among us.

Scott Peck makes the point that our nature is defined by process in this paraphrase of T. H. White's parable of the embryo in *The Sword and the Stone*:

> ...it was back in the very early days, when all of the earth's creatures were still in embryonic form. God called all the little embryos together one afternoon and said: "I'm going to give each of you whatever three things you want. So come up here one by one and ask for whatever three things you want and I will give them to you."
>
> So the first little embryo came up and said, "God, I'd like to have hands and feet in the shape of spades so I can dig myself a safe home underneath the ground, and I'd like to have a thick, furry coat to keep me warm in the winter, and I would like to have some sharp front teeth so I can chew on the grasses."
>
> And God said, "Fine, go and be a woodchuck."
>
> Then the next little embryo came up and said, "God, what I like is the water, and I'd like to have a flexible body so I can swim around in it. I'd also like to breathe underwater with some kind of gills, and I'd like a system that will keep me warm no matter what the temperature of the water is."
>
> And God said, "Fine, go be a fish."
>
> God went through all the little embryos until there was just one left, which seemed to be a particularly shy little embryo....It was so shy that God had to motion it forward and ask, "All right, last little embryo, what three things would you like?" And it said, "Well, I don't want to seem pre-presumptuous or anything. It's not that I'm not...ah...grateful, because I am. But...but I was wondering if maybe...if it was all right with You...I could stay just the way I am—an embryo. Maybe sometime later when I'm smart enough to know three things I really want, I can ask You for them then...Or maybe...if You want me to become a certain something, You can give me the three things You think I need."
>
> And God smiled and said, "Ah, you are human. And because you have chosen to remain a perpetual embryo, I will give you dominion over all of the other creatures."[3]

Peck's point is this: to be in process is our nature. Again, those who frighten me the most in the church, or in society in general, are those who claim to possess the answers. To me they are the "insane" ones in that they deny their very nature through their conviction that they no longer stand in need of spiritual growth.

Rather than believing that I might someday possess the truth, I believe that all of us are by our very nature like the third embryo in T. H. White's parable. That is, we are always unfinished. To attempt to "finish" ourselves completely on our own without God is "insane" and hurls us headlong into the miseries of this disease and its attendant penchant for idolatry.

Today, because I have decided to believe that God can restore me to sanity, I am very much like the third embryo. Every new day I venture forth to the throne of grace, where I offer words similar to those found in the parable. My prayer goes something like this: "God, I am insane when I make myself God. I am insane when I attempt to finish me. I thank you that I am not yet finished, and I trust you to do that job with me. I will get out of the way and cooperate just today with your divine will. Thank you. Amen."

It is little wonder to me that so many people were spiritually abused in childhood. What I believe occurs so often in the context of such spiritual abuse is that someone attempts to "finish" other folks by shoving some amorphous perception of a truth down their throats. Such an imposition is not only spiritual abuse, it is insanity.

Flannery O'Connor illustrates this kind of abuse eloquently in "The Enduring Chill." In one scene there is an encounter between a dying young writer and an Irish priest who comes to the dying man's bed in preparation for the last rites. The writer, though not a Christian, invites the priest to his bedside because the young man longs for sympathy from a cultured man who might fully appreciate the tragedy of his untimely death. He had hoped for a Jesuit; instead he gets an aging, rigid Irish priest.

The absurd scene begins with the writer, Asbury Fox, inquiring of the priest his opinions regarding James Joyce:

> *The priest brushed his huge hand in the air as if he were bothered by gnats. "I haven't met him [James Joyce]," he said. "Now. Do you say your morning prayers and night prayers?"*
>
> *Asbury appeared confused. "Joyce was a great writer," he murmured ...*
>
> *"You don't eh," said the priest. "Well, you will never learn to be good unless you pray regularly. You cannot love Jesus unless you speak to Him."*
>
> *"The myth of the dying god has always fascinated me," Asbury shouted, but the priest did not appear to catch it.*
>
> *"Do you have trouble with purity?" he demanded, and as Asbury paled, he went on without waiting for an answer. "We all do but you must pray to the Holy Ghost for it. Mind, heart, and body. Nothing is overcome without prayer. Pray with your family. Do you pray with your family?"*
>
> *"God forbid," Asbury answered. "My mother doesn't have time to*

Step 2: God can restore me to sanity.

pray and my sister is an atheist," he shouted.

"A shame!" said the priest. *"Then you must pray for them."*

"An artist prays by creating," Asbury ventured.

"Not enough!" snapped the priest. *"If you do not pray daily, you are neglecting your immortal soul. Do you know your catechism?"*

"Certainly not," Asbury muttered.

"Who made you?" the priest asked in a martial tone.

"Different people believe different things about that," Asbury said.

"God made you," the priest said shortly. *"Who is God?"*

"God is an idea created by man," Asbury said, feeling that he was getting into stride, that two could play at this.

"God is spirit infinitely perfect," the priest said. *"You are very ignorant boy. Why did God make you?"*

"God didn't ..."

"God made you to know Him, to love Him, to serve Him in this world, and to be happy with Him in the next!" the old priest said in a battering voice. *"If you don't apply yourself to the catechism, how do you expect to save your immortal soul?"*

Asbury saw he had made a mistake and that it was time to get rid of the old fool. *"Listen,"* he said. *"I'm not a Roman."*

"A poor excuse for not saying your prayers!" the old man snorted.

Asbury slumped slightly in the bed. *"I'm dying,"* he shouted.

"But you are not dead yet!" said the priest... . *"God does not send the Holy Ghost to those who don't ask Him. Ask Him to send the Holy Ghost."*

"The Holy Ghost?" Asbury said.

"Are you so ignorant that you've never heard of the Holy Ghost?" the priest asked.

"Certainly I've heard of the Holy Ghost," Asbury said furiously, *"and the Holy Ghost is the last thing I am looking for!"*

"And he may be the last thing you get," the priest said...[4]

Flannery O'Connor's dialogue between the Irish priest and the writer represents a head-on collision between two idolaters. Idolaters? How could that be? One is obviously a man of faith who, though a bit intrusive and quite insensitive, is up to nothing more grievous than working within the constructs of his own, perhaps narrow, doctrines to "save" a man's soul.

From my perspective, both men have missed, overlooked, or abandoned the fundamental truth that we, all of us, are *always* in the process that is illustrated magnificently in the parable of the embryos.

The priest has come to idolize his doctrines. Long ago he gave up thinking and savoring the process of discovering his own truth. And what about Asbury? Even though I find him to be the more appealing of the two characters in this tense drama, I also view him as an idolater. He has long idolized his skepticism and, if you will, seems to have swapped his craft for any kind of authentic journey into his own soul. In my view, artistic expression can be very safe if it does not emanate from one's own awareness of a deeply wounded soul.

Read again the impasse contained in the priest's frustration with Asbury: "If you don't apply yourself to the catechism, how do you expect to save your immortal soul?" When I first read this story, I recall being simply frustrated. As I have read it again in the context of recovery, I am struck by the insanity of the situation it describes. You see, the priest's primary tenet—that we can somehow come to know how to save our own immortal souls—flies in the face of most everything I have come to accept as truth through my program of working the 12 Steps. Unlike the priest's position that a body of knowledge can save my immortal soul, I have come to believe that I am wholly powerless over the issue of my own salvation. God is not powerless over that question, but I certainly am. I have no doubt about that. Further, I have come to believe that knowledge will not save me, or anything or anyone else, for that matter. But I now recognize, because I have practiced Step 2 for years, that God's grace can, has, and will continue to save me.

For me to adopt either the idolatrous fundamentalism of the priest or the rigid skepticism of the writer as my personal faith would quickly make me crazy. And in making myself insane, I am quickly at odds with the principle of the 2nd Step, which maintains that I have come to believe that God (as revealed in Jesus Christ) can restore me to sanity. My theological convictions, no matter how sound and well thought out, cannot restore me to much of anything except the illusion of self-satisfaction. And my own critical projections regarding any particular systematic doctrine are totally useless to me in the context of the saving of my life, soul, sanity, or anything else.

Asbury and the priest missed each other because they failed to love. The entire episode occurred beneath the banner of a faith in a God, which I suspect both men believed had something to do with what it means to love. But the problem revealed in this story is that neither man knew, or had any real experience with, what it meant to love. Hence, in my view, both were "insane."

Some years ago, I experienced a similarly sad moment in my own ministry in Dallas. It was Lent, and our senior pastor, my immediate supervisor, invited me to lead a Bible study at the posh North Dallas home of a

Step 2: God can restore me to sanity.

couple who were members of our church. According to the pastor's plan, these folks were to invite church members who resided in their area to their home for a study of Paul's Letter to the Church at Ephesus.

My hosts for the evening were, in my view, more than a little rigid in their convictions about the faith. I had been instructed by a friend, a colleague, to soft-pedal some of my theological convictions, such as my adamant agreement with Paul that "God's power is made perfect in weakness."[5]

Our evening began smoothly. The host couple seemed glad enough to welcome me into their home. Other folks, about twenty in all, joined us for the Bible study. One talented woman accompanied us on a piano as we sang some old favorites from a hymnal with which I was not at all familiar.

Following our final hymn, the hostess offered what I sensed was a very sincere prayer. She turned to me at the conclusion of her own "amen," and I fully expected her to invite me to begin the study of Ephesians. Instead she surprised, even stunned me with this stern question. "Are you saved?" she asked me with a beatific smile growing across her tense face.

I said, "I don't know for certain. If I did know that for certain, then my guess is that I am," I continued. "But you see, that issue is up to God and to God alone. For me to answer in place of God would be, at the very least, presumptuous."

Suffice it to say that today, in the wake of my experience with recovery, I would have answered the question quite differently. If I were to be asked the same question today, my answer would be simply, "Yes. One day at a time."

But I introduced the woman to my own uncertainty as well as to my unwillingness to be presumptuous in the presence of God, and she was both angry and deeply disappointed. She rose from the comfortable love seat she shared with her, I assume, equally disappointed husband and offered the following painful pronouncement: "I cannot believe that one of my pastors does not know whether or not he is saved. Please leave."

I was shaken and more hurt than angry. (The anger arrived days later.) I offered no word of argument, reached down and picked up my Bible, and made the most dignified exit that I could manage under the difficult circumstances.

I believe now that like Asbury and the priest in Flannery O'Connor's tale the hostess and I were both wrong in that unwittingly we had, both of us, become idolaters.

In seminary I instructed myself well to worship at the throne of the sophisticated questions. At some very different place, this woman, who regarded herself as a very pious Christian, learned to worship, I suspect, at the throne of pat answers and a black-and-white, literal, view of reality.

Such subtle idolatry transports us, I am convinced, to the very threshold of insanity. Why? Because it delivers us to disappointment. My sophisticated, seminary-trained thinking cannot restore me to sanity, just as the woman's rigid religious ideologies will never bring her the peace she claims, I presume, to seek so diligently.

Step 2 says that I have come to believe that a Higher Power (and again, as a Christian, I say God as revealed in Jesus Christ) can restore me to sanity. As soon as I place my faith anywhere other than in God, I get into trouble and begin the slow slide toward insanity.

As I was writing this book, one of my heroes visited me. His name is Andy, and he is an octogenarian who for decades made an enormous contribution to the Kingdom of God as the president of small college.

Andy "interrupted" my writing to tell me with prodigious vigor of his ministry to the maximum-security block at the state penitentiary. Once a month he travels to this cell block to teach the Word of God to men who have been convicted of murder and rape. In Andy's words, "My Bible students ain't in there because they tilted no pinball machine."

After more than seven years, close to two hundred men in this maximum-security unit assemble each month to hear Andy teach the Word of God. They have come to trust and to love this humble, gifted man of God. On one such visit, he was summoned to the "Death Cell," which is a primitive hospice where the incarcerated are taken when they are judged by the hospital physicians to have no more than two weeks to live. Most of the men in the Death Cell are dying from AIDS, but the man who summoned Andy that Sunday evening was suffering from the early demise of both kidneys.

The dying man, an African American of about fifty-five, waved at him feebly from a wheelchair. Andy bent forward, and the dying inmate whispered to him in a voice so ravaged by disease as to be hardly audible, "Andy, I have two weeks to live. I want to sing in the prison choir one more time. Would you pray to God that I might have that request granted? I want to live one more month just so that I can sing once more in the prison choir."

Andy no doubt disappointed the man when he waved his head in the sure direction of "No." He then looked the convict squarely in the eyes and whispered, "Look, you pray for yourself. God knows you as well as God knows me. Besides, I'm on God's back all the time, and there is no

Step 2: God can restore me to sanity.

doubt in my mind that I pray so often that most of my petitions get mixed up with the Rotarians' invocations."

Andy shook the man's hand and departed. A month later the man showed up to sing in the prison choir. He had been dismissed from the Death Cell. All that the doctors had written in their official reports was that one of the man's kidneys had begun to function again.

I peered into Andy's clear blue eyes and I asked, "How would that story play out in most mainline churches or even at our so-called liberal seminaries?" He smiled slightly and spoke what I regard to be the truth: "The church and most seminaries would not understand it."

I am afraid he is right. And before my own recovery I would have scoffed at it. Perhaps the kidney did just choose to begin functioning. I don't know because I am not God. But I am witness to similar healing in my own life as well as in the lives of countless folks who have learned what it means to experience serenity when they have never before known even a moment's peace. In my own perspective, such healing, which brings a person from chaos to serenity, is every bit as impressive as a kidney that decides on its on to begin functioning again even after all manner of standard medical procedures have failed.

So I no longer scoff at God's power to heal. I am living, breathing evidence of God's grace. But the fact is that I do despair in the wake of my subjective impression that this culture's religious institutions are all too often as idolatrous in their own subtle, sophisticated, and culturally sanctioned manners as were those folks who long ago danced around a golden calf on a warm desert night.

You see, every human being, every single one of us, yearns for God. Whether it is the pope or some inmate in the Texas Department of Corrections, the fact is that all of us yearn for God. But only one of our problems with this yearning is that, through our penchant for organization, most of us have replaced God altogether with institutions. Consequently, we have equated the mystery of God with our creeds, doctrines, polities, traditions, customs, folkways, and particular denominational entities. And in this unhealthy equation, we have displaced God from the center of our lives rather than depending on the only force powerful enough to heal us and, ultimately, to save us.

Am I opposed to organized religion? Of course not! I am, however, adamantly opposed to the equation of our institutions with holiness. And in my view, those of us who compose the mainline church are very guilty of the sin of displacement.

Gerald May writes of our yearning for God:

After twenty years of listening to the yearnings of people's hearts,

I am convinced that all human beings have an inborn desire for God. Whether we are consciously religious or not, this desire is our deepest longing and our most precious treasure. It gives us meaning. Some of us have repressed this desire, burying it beneath so many other interests that we are completely unaware of it. Or we may experience it in different ways—as a longing for wholeness, completion, or fulfillment. Regardless of how we describe it, it is a longing for love... This yearning is the essence of the human spirit, it is the origin of our highest hopes and most noble dreams.[6]

Twenty-six hundred years before Gerald May, another writer, this one a Hebrew prophet by the name of Isaiah, penned what I regard to be a very similar message (Isa. 44:12–19):

The iron smith fashions it and works it over the coals; he shapes it with hammer and forges it with his strong arm; he becomes hungry and his strength fails, he drinks no water and he is faint. The carpenter stretches a line, he marks it out with a pencil; he fashions it with planes, and marks it with a compass; he shapes it into the figure of a man, with the beauty of a man, to dwell in a house. He cuts down cedars; or he chooses a holm tree or an oak and lets it grow strong among the trees of the forest; he plants a cedar and rain nourishes it. Then it becomes fuel for a man; he takes a part of it and warms himself; also he makes a god and worships it, he makes it a graven image and falls down before it. Half of it he burns in the fire; over the half he eats flesh, he roasts meat and is satisfied; also he warms himself and says, "Aha, I am warm, I have seen the fire!" And the rest of it he makes into a god, his idol; and falls down to it and worships it; he prays to it and says "Deliver me, for thou art my god!"

They know not, nor do they discern; for he has shut their eyes so that they cannot see, and their minds, so that they cannot understand. No one considers, nor is there knowledge or discernment to say "Half of it I burned in the fire, I also baked bread on its coals, I roasted flesh and have eaten; and shall I make a residue of it an abomination? Shall I fall down before a block of wood?"[7]

This question posed by a prophet twenty-six hundred years ago is today our question, as well. "Shall I fall down to a block of wood?" You and I, like the characters in Isaiah's poetic depiction of humanity, yearn for God. Whether we are conscious of it or not, this yearning for God is our deepest longing, Gerald May informs us. And yet, all too often what the process of displacement has made us make of our "God experience" in this culture is nothing more than one more block of wood.

Step 2: God can restore me to sanity.

You and I cannot be saved by a block of wood. Neither can we be saved by any particular creed. I cannot be restored to sanity by any one doctrine. No denomination, no matter how sincere, can bring me to the point of personal salvation. Not even the most dedicated group of 12 Steppers can bring me to a place of peace. Only God can do that. And this is precisely what the 2nd Step states. I have come to believe that *God*, not anything or anyone else, no matter how sacred the institution, can restore me to sanity.

In the course of long conversations with contemporary theologian Matthew Fox, Lawrence Wright recorded what Fox describes as the five boulders that block, or impede, us from enjoying the kind of relationship with God that can restore us to sanity. The first of those boulders is acedia. This, according to Fox, is a medieval term that means "depression," but that also encompasses the sins of sloth, cynicism, and pessimism. He reminds us that Thomas Aquinas defines acedia as a sluggishness of the mind that quite simply neglects being good. Acedia is marked by a preoccupation with death. "Where is the vitality," Matthew Fox asks, "in our political, economic and educational systems?" From Fox's perspective, depression is not just a personal psychological issue, but a cultural or collective state into which we have slipped.

I believe that he is correct. Often I ask people who come to see me if they have peace in their lives. The answer is almost always a ringing "No!"

Fox's second boulder is apathy. He informs us that *apathy* comes from the contraction of two Greek words that together mean "no passion." This boulder is best described by our failure, or by our unwillingness, to love. When we are apathetic about our own lives, and when we fail to love ourselves, we are setting ourselves up for an inevitable sense of overwhelming despair.

The third boulder is addiction. For me, this term is synonymous with idolatry. According to Fox, addiction keeps us from knowing our inner selves in that it dissuades us from sojourning in the soul, where authentic recovery invariably calls us.

The fourth boulder is anthropocentrism. This is a five-dollar word for the bias toward interpreting everything in terms of human beings. What I suspect he means to convey here is that, through our anthropocentric perspective of "reality," we naturally tend to limit our view of God and God's power. In that we readily recognize that we do not know love all that well, by viewing God through an anthropocentric lens, we come to believe that God is just as limited as we are in what it means to love. Nothing could be farther from the truth, of course. God's love and God's power to heal us far exceed any reality or any experience that we might ever imagine.

The final boulder is avarice. The greed for gain, in Fox's perspective, knows no limit and tends toward infinity. In my view, avarice is nothing more than another form of displacement. We displace our spiritual quest for God with our insatiable quest for things, symbols, and the illusion of security.[8]

My grandfather taught me that, if you can't go *through* something, go around it. One of the beautiful truths of the 2nd Step is that it does just that. It sidesteps all five of Matthew Fox's impediments to the spiritual life. If I truly come to believe that a Higher Power (for me, God as revealed in Jesus Christ) can restore me to sanity, then I take a step in faith out of my depression. My experience, therefore, with personal acedia is behind me.

There can be no place for apathy in the 2nd Step in that this Step, like all of the 12 Steps, is a move; it is an action that is, by definition, the very antithesis of apathy. Step 2 is designed to liberate me from my addictions; therefore, boulder number three, addiction, also loses its power in my life. I am no longer in the business of displacing God, but I now live a life of what I term "replacement." Simply put, I have replaced a god with God.

Immediately as I move into the 2nd Step I encounter mystery, and mystery, of course, can never be viewed through the lens of anthropocentrism. Mystery, by its very nature demands sovereignty. I cannot control mystery. If I could, it would not be a mystery. I can only accept it for what it is. And through faith, I have come to believe that a mystery is far more powerful than I, and that it can and will restore me to sanity. Therefore, Matthew Fox's fourth boulder is also sidestepped.

As I continue to practice Step 2, I reorient my priorities dramatically. Sanity, for me, means, as I mentioned at the outset of this chapter, is reflected in the life of Jesus as it is recorded in the New Testament. What I have discovered in the life, ministry, death, and resurrection of Jesus is a man who warned repeatedly against building loftier barns to accumulate treasure where it might be consumed by fire or moths.

In the course of my own recovery I have come to view Fox's fifth boulder, avarice, as nothing more than an archaic defense mechanism for my raging fear. Once again, the 2nd Step is terribly profound in that it grounds me again and again in the incontrovertible truth that it is God, as opposed to any object of my greed, that can restore me to sanity.

I've tried the idols and found them wanting. "No, thank you," I say daily to greed. And the honest truth is that I must say it at least that

Step 2: God can restore me to sanity.

often, because of the five boulders in Matthew Fox's mind, the fifth is by far the most difficult for me. From the look of things in this culture, I suspect that I am not alone in struggling with what it means to be greedy.

I have decided to conclude this chapter concerning Step 2 with an anecdote from my decade of ministry on the streets of Dallas with the homeless. During the course of that work, I came to know a large, imposing, athletically built young man who appeared to me to be both sensitive and highly intelligent. I will call him John.

John is an alcoholic. On his more-sober-than-drunk days he would stumble into our church basement soup kitchen and more or less behave himself. On those days, however, when he was more inebriated than sane, we would bar him from even entering the front door of the soup kitchen.

I noticed one morning that John had been absent from the soup kitchen for some time. As fate or, far more likely, God would have it, an ornery little street character named Billy tapped on my office door the very next morning to inform me that John was lying "dead" beneath an abandoned icehouse in South Dallas.

I solicited the help of a priest, who was my dear friend, and this man and I drove a church van to the icehouse. John lay beneath the pier-and-beam foundation unconscious, but, thankfully, he had not yet succumbed to death. He was very sick and had crawled under the icehouse to die. His plan was as simple as it was horrific: he would simply drink himself to death there.

Very gently, the priest and I rolled his enormous body onto a wool blanket, and then with great care we dragged John from the shadows into the bright light of the new morning. For the first time I heard him offer a loud groan as he struggled to open his eyes.

Our journey in the church van to Parkland Hospital proved uneventful. Once inside the hospital, with John securely strapped to a stainless steel gurney, I paused long enough to inform the attending physician of what I am certain he had already surmised. "John," I said, "is a drunk. If he drinks much more alcohol, he is a dead man."

Three weeks later, John shuffled again into the soup kitchen. This time his face was as emaciated as it was somber. I invited him into my small office, and I will never forget his story. He informed me that some time during his "incarceration," as he termed his hospitalization, he made a conscious decision to live. He reported that the hospital room immediately filled with a light so intense that it blinded him even more than the sun had done on the morning that the priest and I pulled him from under the icehouse.

In that brightness he discovered both an external warmth and a peace that he had never before experienced. Then he said, "Bob, I didn't even know how to pray. But I reckon that is exactly what I did. Because I said to that light, 'I want to live.'"

He did recover, and today he holds a very responsible position with a church-sponsored nonprofit corporation that ministers quite efficaciously to homeless men and women.

John did not know at the moment of his experience with grace even one utterance of the 12 Steps. The fact is that he did not need to know even a syllable of these Steps. That is just one of the beauties of this miraculous discipline. God will never permit us to make of these Steps an institution or another set of 12 flashy new idols we can cling to in hopes of finding our salvation.

We do not have to utter the words in any particular way or under any unique set of circumstances. We don't have to get them in the "right" order. All that is required of us for healing is that we ask to be restored to sanity. John simply said, "I want to live." In my mind, those words were his 2nd Step. In uttering those four words, this good man was, in fact, and wholly unbeknownst even to himself, taking Step 2. Some time following his release from the hospital, he spoke the words of Step 1, and since that day his life has not been the same. To God goes the glory for John's discovery of what it means to be sane.

Any step toward restoration is invariably a step toward God. Nothing else is powerful enough to restore us to sanity. It is that basic—and that simple. It is also very difficult, if not impossible, to comprehend. Give up attempting to understand Step 2. Simply work it, and it will work for you.

References

[1] Lawrence Wright, *Saints and Sinners* (New York: Knopf, 1993), p. 243.

[2] M. Scott Peck, *Further along the Road Less Traveled* (New York: Simon and Schuster, 1993), p. 160.

[3] Ibid., pp. 117–118.

[4] Flannery O'Connor, *The Complete Stories* (New York: Farrar, Strauss and Giroux, 1971), pp. 375–377.

[5] 2 Cor. 12:9 RSV.

[6] Gerald May, *Addiction and Grace* (New York: Harper and Row, 1988), p. 1.

[7] Isaiah 44:12–19 RSV.

[8] Lawrence Wright, pp. 243–244.

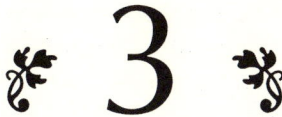

Put off your old nature which belongs to your former manner of life and is corrupt through deceitful lusts, and be renewed in the spirit of your minds, and put on the new nature, created after the likeness of God in true righteousness and holiness.

Ephesians 4:22–24 RSV

Step 3: *I turn my will and my life over to the care of God as I understand God.*

Some months ago I was listening to a man being interviewed by Dr. Gerald Mann on his nationally syndicated television talk show. The gentleman offered Dr. Mann the following summation of the first three Steps:

> Step 1: I can't.
> Step 2: God can.
> Step 3: I'll let him.

Sounds easy enough, doesn't it? Well, don't be fooled. Step 3 is very, very difficult. It is what I have learned to call the "Surrender" Step. Surrender is not easy, especially if you're an American male nurtured both physically and spiritually in the Piney Woods of East Texas not more than twenty miles from a natural spring where Davy Crockett and his band of Tennessee adventurers camped on their trek to the Alamo. With that kind of heritage, surrender is not in my vocabulary, and neither does it flow in my bloodline.

No matter how difficult surrender might be, it is the path to serenity. The predicate to surrender is, of course, faith. I must have faith that there is something out there in the void to which I can surrender.

In the context of my own recovery the following quote by the French moralist La Rochefoucauld encourages me in the direction of what it means to surrender: "...one might say that just as the small fire is extinguished by the storm whereas a large fire is enhanced by it—likewise a weak faith is weakened by predicaments and catastrophes whereas a strong faith is strengthened by them."[1] In a very real sense the "fires" this disease brings on us can, if we allow them to do so, actually strengthen our faith.

Consistently, I hear folks in recovery meetings express their gratitude for the disease. "Were it not for my alcoholism, or codependency, or sex addiction, I would never have discovered grace," they offer without even a hint of humiliation. If we allow these addictions negative power in our lives, the catastrophes we experience will tear us down every time. But if we reframe the difficulties, as well as the catastrophes, and begin to view them through the spiritual lens of recovery, we will quickly come to discover that our problems, yes, even our catastrophes, are nothing less than God's marvelous gifts of grace.

It is truly amazing to me that the 12 Steps have survived, even flourished, in a culture so influenced by the psychoanalytic view introduced in the writings of Sigmund Freud. Thank God, there were several brilliant post-Freudian writers and thinkers, among them Viktor Frankl, who introduced spirituality into the disciplines of mental health. To Freud, the ego (or one's conscious sense of self) was regarded as, ultimately, the plaything of the unconscious drives. Freud once wrote that the ego is not the master of its own house.[2]

I view my ego, in the context of this particular theory, as what in East Texas we used to call a "fishing cork." When I was a kid we would toss a fishing cork, unattached to any line, hook, or sinker, upon the murky water of a stock tank so that we might watch with delight as the sunfish and cherry gills swam to the surface to bump it around and more or less have their way with it. In Freud's theory, as evaluated by Viktor Frankl, "psychological phenomena are reduced to drives and instincts and thus seem to be totally determined by them—determined in the sense of cause and effect."[3] If it is true that our ego is nothing more than some fishing cork being pushed around by what lies beneath the surface, then Step 3 remains wholly impossible. Therefore, anyone would be wise to back off

Step 3: I turn my life over to God.

from this Step and declare in a voice louder than a braying jackass on the hungry side of the fence that the entire program of recovery is nothing but one bogus enterprise preying upon the hurting and the gullible.

Try peddling that belief, though, to the millions of alcoholics and addicts who have experienced healing and who have come to know the first genuine peace they have ever experienced. I can tell you that not one of those folks will claim that they are driven entirely and exclusively by the unconscious drives that are so fundamental to Freud's psychoanalytic theory. To Freud, being human was interpreted to mean being driven.[4] Those of us, however, who have practiced these 12 Steps of healing would, I believe, offer a radically different view of what it means to be human. I suspect that we would say something like this: being human means being free. We are free to remain stuck in our disease and eventually to allow it to kill us, or we are free, in the words of Jesus Christ, to have life and to have it abundantly.

Viktor Frankl saw early on in his development as a respected theoretician and practitioner the *absolute* necessity of including the spiritual dimension in any discussion of mental and emotional healing. When Frankl employs the term "spiritual," he is doing so without any religious connotation; rather, what he intends to communicate through the word is what he terms "a specifically human phenomenon." Succinctly, for Frankl the "spiritual" is that dimension that is human in a man or a woman. In other words, it is that part of us that makes us uniquely human.[5]

To Frankl, a "spiritual phenomenon" may be conscious or unconscious. The spiritual basis of human existence, however, is ultimately unconscious. Therefore, the center of the human person is unconscious. In its origin, the human spirit must be regarded as unconscious spirit.[6]

To couch this theory in a language that is simple but, I hope, not simplistic, what Frankl is offering us is a departure from the traditional psychoanalytic (Freudian) view. As opposed to our core's being viewed as comprising drives that control us (Freud's view), we are, in fact, at our very core one unconscious essence—spirit. We are not conscious of this spiritual essence, of course, but it is this spiritual quality that differentiates us from other living beings. Again, keep in mind that this core spiritual essence is unconscious and therefore wholly beyond our awareness.

Frankl provides us with a far better illustration than any I might dredge up:

> *This [our awareness of the spiritual core] is not unlike the eye—precisely at the place of its origin the retina has its "blind spot," as the entrance of the optical nerve is called in anatomy. Likewise, the*

> *spirit is blind precisely where it has its origin—precisely there no self observation, no mirroring of itself is possible; where the spirit is "original spirit," where it is fully itself, precisely there it is unconscious of itself.*[7]

What Viktor Frankl has given to us is a very important insight into our humanity that stretches far beyond the formerly, and generally, accepted, perception that we human beings are mere machines driven by internal forces beyond our control. His view is radically different. He sees us not as the playthings of drives, but as spiritual beings bumping around in this existence and waiting to discover the ultimate truth of our own essence, that is, of our own spirituality.

If Freud had been right, that is, if the human sense of self could be degraded to a mere epiphenomenon, then no program of spiritual recovery would have proved in any way efficacious.[8] But Freud was wrong, dead wrong.

To understand the relationship between your own unconscious spirituality and God, contemplate your own navel. (I've been accused of doing that by many of my critics over the years.) According to Frankl, the human navel can be understood only in the context of personal history, for it points beyond the individual to the origin of his or her mother. When I look at my navel I quite naturally see a connection to my own mother, or, if you will, to my earthly origins.

The same is true with the conscience, or with our sense of morality, of right and wrong. It can be fully understood only as pointing to its own transcendent origin. Our conscience maintains a key position in disclosing to us the essential transcendence of the spiritual unconscious.[9]

The best place I know to view this relationship among conscience, transcendence, and spiritual unconscious is in the Old Testament story of Samuel:

> *When Samuel was a boy, he once spent a night in the temple with the high priest Eli. He was awakened by a voice calling him by name. He rose and asked Eli what he wanted; but the high priest had not called him and told him to go back to sleep. The same thing happened a second time, and only when it happened a third time did the high priest tell the boy that the next time he heard his name called, he should stand up and say, "Speak Lord; for thy servant heareth."*[10]

Frankl employs this story from the Old Testament to make the following point: the conscience, that is, our sense of morality, not only refers to transcendence, it originates in transcendence.[11] Is this tantamount to suggesting that we are created in the image of God, as is proclaimed in Genesis? I cannot, of course, speak for Frankl, but to me that is pre-

Step 3: I turn my life over to God.

cisely the point. I cannot surrender myself to myself. No, I must surrender to something higher than myself, and Frankl's immeasurable contribution to twentieth-century thinking on what it means to be mentally healthy, or whole, is that he inextricably links the human unconscious as well as our conscience to that reality we know as God.

In more theological language, the point he makes is that God (transcendence) is both immanent and transcendent. Therefore, in Frankl's words, the self can never be its own lawgiver. It simply cannot issue any categorical imperative because the categorical imperative can come only from the transcendent.[12]

In my own very simple, backwoods way of viewing such complexity, I think what Viktor Frankl has given us is a high-powered way of stating a truth those of us in recovery have long embraced: you and I *must* surrender to something higher than ourselves, simply because we have not been able to make our lives work.

When I was a kid working on a ranch in Colorado, I had a date one moonlit night with a young woman who, it turns out, was from one of the wealthiest families in all of Denver. Her parents had invited me to join them for an evening of Opera in the Park. It was, I am certain, one mighty fine opera. I did make the mistake of asking my date at the intermission if this was the "half-time." It took little time for me to discover that this young debutante's parents were not impressed by a Texas boy whose college mascot was a kangaroo.

Following the opera, I drove the young woman in my (according to Ralph Nader) "unsafe at any speed" Corvair to her parents' mansion. By the time I caught the lights of Denver flickering in my rearview mirror, it was close to midnight.

Suddenly I realized that I was terribly sleepy. Both the opera and this woman's parents had combined to form an effective sedative. I searched for a fast food place where I might purchase a cup of black coffee. I could locate no such establishments open on the outskirts of Boulder. Therefore, I turned my little car in the direction of Lyons, Colorado, and it was in that quaint hamlet nestled in the red rocks of the foothills that I spotted a neon Coors beer sign flashing in the darkness.

I parked on the gravel driveway, popped open the Corvair's front door, climbed the rock steps, and pulled open the door to an otherwise ordinary roadside tavern. The young man behind the bar glanced up from his obvious dedication to the task of drying a hundred or more glasses and said, "Sorry, mister, we're closed."

"I just wondered if I could buy a quick cup of coffee," I asked.

"Sure, come in. I'll give you one," he answered. He sat across from me in silence as I sipped the first taste. It was then that I began to study words that were obviously hand-carved into an imposing log hanging by logging chains against the mirror immediately behind the bar:

> Fear pounded on my door.
> Faith answered . . .
> And no one was there.

I thought it rather odd that such a curious proverb would be hanging in a roadhouse. When I questioned the young bartender regarding the words, he answered, "I don't know the origin of those words. But I heard them often enough when I was in 'Nam. They kept me going. I'm not a religious person, but somehow they comforted me."

I arose from my place at the bar and thanked the young man for his kindness. I have pondered for close to thirty years now the words he carved on the trunk of a lodge pole pine.

In my estimation, what the young veteran had discovered, whether he was alcoholic or not, was the very essence of Step 3. For certainly pain has pounded on my door for the whole of my life. Finally, and only because I knew of nowhere else to turn, I turned to my faith. I answered the door, and the pain, in time, vanished.

In a very real sense, by working the 3rd Step I finally came home to the God who created me as well as to the spirit who dwells within my unconscious being. This, in my subjective view, is precisely why the 3rd Step works: it returns me simultaneously to myself as well as to the one who created me, and who, I believe longs to redeem me.

Thomas Merton writes, "There is a natural desire for heaven, for the fruition of God in us."[13] In my perspective, it is this very "naturalness" that is fundamental for Step 3 ever to prove efficacious in the life of any human being. Surrender *never* feels natural. And I believe that this is because the culture has indoctrinated us effectively, and to our detriment, to avoid what it means to surrender in much the same way we avoid the measles or any other contagious disease. Surrender is considered weak, soft, and, at best, humiliating.

But the cultural indoctrination is a lie. The vast majority of the messages the culture bestows upon us are just flat wrong. There is no other way to say it. Surrender is exactly that which Thomas Merton terms the expression of our *natural* desire for the fruition of God in us.[14] To me, this is a simple, but terribly profound, reiteration of what Frankl is writing about when he inextricably links the spiritual unconscious to the transcendent.

The culture lied to me for the whole of my life, and I suspect that it has lied to you as well. Here are just some of the lies it taught me. Be perfect. Be strong. Never make mistakes. Deny your failures. Shame yourself often. Find all manner of weaknesses in your brothers and sisters and judge them harshly and regularly. Strive always to be the best. It doesn't matter whether you succeed or fail, as long as you do your best. Winning is not everything; it is the only thing. Never fail! Humiliate the weak, the foolish, the stupid among you, but never humiliate yourself. Never show them your weaknesses. Never confess to being wrong. Grab for all the pleasure you can get. You only go around once. Use things as well as people. And finally, go to church regularly. It's good for business.

The culture lied, and I bought it whole hog. Today, I accept full responsibility for the lies that I ingested, digested, and then struggled to live on. It is not the culture's fault; it is my responsibility. But the fact remains that the culture is a powerful purveyor of "untruth." For decades, and until that gift of grace I now know as my symbols of depression and anxiety shepherded me toward Step 3, I was swimming, more accurately, drowning, in an ocean of lies.

Even though I have been instructed by the culture in a fundamental untruth to the contrary, my natural desire was then, and is today, *always* for God. It is the same with all of us, whether we know it or not, or whether or not we admit it.

I very much like the way in which Gerald May writes about what Thomas Merton terms our "natural desire for heaven":

God created us to seek God, with the hope that we might grope after God through the shadows of our ignorance . . .

From a psychoanalytic perspective one could say that we displace our longing for God upon other things; we cathect them instead of God....

Perhaps our displacement of desire for God makes sense from God's perspective as well. After all, it is God who created us with our propensity for addiction....

What would happen to our freedom if God, our perfect lover, were to appear before us with such objective clarity that all of our doubts disappeared? We would experience a kind of love to be sure, but it would be love like a reflex. Almost without thought, we would fix all our desires upon this Divine Object, try to grasp it and possess it, addict ourselves to it.

I think God refuses to be the object of our attachment because God desires full love and not addiction. Love born of freedom...requires that we search for a deepening awareness of God.....True love, then, is not only born of freedom; but is born also of difficult choice.[15]

In my view, Step 3 is the difficult choice to which May alludes. It is clearly the choice of God over what May characterizes as "other goodnesses," or what I term "other gods."

Thomas Merton is so right when he tells us, "Our minds are like crows. They pick up everything that glitters, no matter how uncomfortable our nests get with all that metal in them."[16] That is a very apt description of my life. I grew up in a Christian family and, from the beginning, I was nurtured in the faith as it was to be found in the old Southern Presbyterian Church. In truth, it was as good a place as any to be nurtured in the faith, and the vast majority of those who taught me in the church were "truth tellers."

I was introduced to God in the church, but still I was tempted to chase after other gods, and I chased after them with a vengeance. But the truth is that I never framed the objects of my attachment and addiction as gods. No, I viewed them as simply the stuff of life, I suppose, as opposed to seeing them for what they were and are—the conscious objects of my obeisance.

In retrospect, though, I can see that they were nothing less than gods, and they had tempted me with a passion. Like some naïve rube, I succumbed regularly to their siren songs without even a shred of awareness that I had swapped the faith of my childhood for worship at the thrones of false gods. I must confess, however, that when I attended church, or even more, when I assisted in the leadership of worship at the First Presbyterian Church of Dallas, I sometimes wondered, but never out loud, why it was that I felt so consistently rotten on the inside when the God I proclaimed from the pulpit and read about in the Scripture and creeds was characterized as the God of peace.

I never made the connection between my own temptation by and capitulation to false gods and my personal misery. None of this even remotely approached my awareness until I began to work the 12 Steps.

This is an ideal place to weave in yet another story of conscious temptation that occurred following my entry into recovery. I offer it as a parable of sorts in that the sad, tragic actually, protagonist in this story has become for me a symbol, or a benchmark, of my lifetime of succumbing both consciously and unconsciously to temptation. Permit me to hasten to add that in this particular context, I did not succumb.

My older brother Bill is, at the time of this writing, among other things, the executive producer of the Dallas Cowboys. That's a high-sounding name given to the position of the person who is responsible for everything that occurs on the Texas Stadium turf other than the actual football contest. This includes the pregame show, the playing or singing of

Step 3: I turn my life over to God.

the National Anthem, the half-time extravaganza, and so forth.

A couple of years ago, my brother graciously invited me to join him at Texas Stadium so that I might watch firsthand, either from the sidelines or from the press box a game between the Cowboys and the Bills.

I gratefully accepted his generous invitation and two hours prior to kick off I wandered to the sidelines acting like I was someone important in the glamorous world of the Dallas Cowboys. During the pregame warm-ups, I heard a young woman calling in a high-pitched voice, "Hey, mister. Hey, mister." Naturally, I glanced up into the stands so that I might discover the source of this lovely, but plaintive, voice. What I discovered was an attractive woman buried in makeup. She waved frenetically as she pointed directly at me.

Once she was satisfied that she had garnered my attention, she scrambled down the aisle and immediately reached for my hand. I took her hand in my own for some reason that had more to do with a cultural reaction than any kind of thought-out response. She then whispered to me this shocking proposal: "I will give you whatever your heart desires if you will just give me your sideline pass."

I was stunned at first and then I felt embarrassment slowly seep into my awareness in the manner well water drips out of a cracked pipe. I struggled to break free from her grip, but this painted lady was not finished and she adamantly refused to let go of my hand. And this time in a loud voice she exclaimed, "I'm talking sex, mister!" She screamed in an even louder voice, "Your all-time fantasies come true!"

I yanked my hand away, smiled at her, and simply said, "No, thank you, ma'am." Suffice it to say that temptation has not often approached me so boldly in such a blatant sexual context, but it presents itself every day of my life in far more subtle and insidious ways. Essentially, its message has consistently come to me in the form of the strong enticement to worship gods other than the God of my creation and the God whose spirit dwells deep in my unconscious.

Temptation is so prevalent in all of our lives and so very real that I am greatly comforted by the inclusion of the fourth chapter of Matthew's Gospel in the canon in that it offers all of us who recognize and do daily battle with temptation the truth that Jesus was also tempted.

Gerald May offers as solid an interpretation as any I've ever read of this episode:

> *Satan suggests that Jesus satisfy his hunger by turning stones into bread. This invitation is remarkably similar to the one the serpent gave to Eve....*
>
> *Failing at this, Satan next tempts Jesus to manipulate God's power*

for the sake of his own self-indulgence, by jumping off the temple parapet. Here the invitation is to test rather than to trust God, to use God superstitiously, as a puppet. Failing once more, Satan proposes the last temptation: he offers Jesus the entire world if he will make Satan his god. This is, of course, the ultimate invitation to idolatry.[17]

It is in the context of this temptation story that I discovered once again the fundamental difference between Jesus and me. Jesus trusted God in that he said "No!" to the Adversary; for the whole of my lifetime I have spoken out of both sides of my mouth in that I have professed trust in God while I have scattered myself to the proverbial four winds chasing after most any god that would have me. Dr. May makes here what I believe is a crucial point when he reminds us that Jesus did not predicate his resistance upon a foundation of his own construction. No, he traveled to a much higher plane. He relied entirely upon the law of God. His words to the Adversary were quotations from Scripture.

To me, Jesus' reliance upon Scripture is prima facie evidence that he was a fully "surrendered" man. It is dangerous, I suppose, to frame Jesus in the twentieth-century garb of our modern-day constructs, but in the context of his own struggle with the Adversary, it is important to note that even he did not try to go it alone. No, he relied upon what he knew. And I have no doubt in my mind that during the first thirty years of his life he studied until he mastered the *Septuagint*, the Greek Old Testament. He knew the law and he stood upon God's law as the essential predicate for the strength necessary to withstand temptation. If Jesus needed God, imagine how foolish it is for you or for me to believe that we can go it alone whenever the Adversary strikes.

As I said earlier, *fear* is my Adversary. It is the power that comes in the night, at the breakfast table, whenever I stand before a group of people to say anything, when I watch my young adult daughter drive off in her small Toyota, and when the bills fall due.

The defense mechanism I have developed over a lifetime of attempts to handle the fear, I term "control." A more clinical definition for the same thing, perhaps, would be "compensation" or "overcompensation." I came to believe that it was my nature to control, when in truth, such a belief was nothing more than a lie. No, my true nature is to trust, but I don't want to do that. I don't find trusting what I cannot see or touch comfortable, but again, the fact is that at some conscious level, I know full well that my controlling behaviors have not served me well, if at all.

Thomas Merton writes, I believe the truth, when he offers: "If I have this divine life in me, what do the accidents of pain and pleasure, hope and fear, joy and sorrow matter to me. They are not my life and have

Step 3: I turn my life over to God.

little to do with it. Why should I fear anything that cannot rob me of God, and why should I desire anything that cannot give me possession of Him?"[18]

I have heard it said that, if a person does not succeed in separating from fear, fear will soon enough separate a person from any awareness of God. The apostle Paul is right, of course, when he writes in Romans 8:35 that nothing can separate us from the love of Christ, but it has been true for me, at least, that my fear has all too often separated me from my own awareness of Christ, or God, in my life.

So how does one get beyond the fear? How does one possibly ever arrive at the place where Thomas Merton obviously was when he wrote, "Why should I fear anything that life cannot rob me of God, and why should I desire anything that cannot give me possession of Him?"[19] The only way I know is to do precisely what Jesus did, that is, to rely entirely upon God when facing the Adversary. And in modern parlance, this is what is commonly termed Step 3. It all has to do with turning our will and our lives over *completely* to the care of God, as we understand God.

I call it surrender, and I know this Step to be the most difficult of the 12. None of them are easy, but this, for me, at least is the real mud hole where I all too often get my own bald tires stuck and where I spin helplessly until my engine begins to smoke.

Again, surrender is very, very difficult in this culture. All of us have been lied to for a lifetime by a culture that offers a panoply of enticing and seductive gods ready, willing, and *temporarily* able to assuage all manner of existential pain. One of the best ways, I suppose, to describe this phenomenon known as surrender, if the mystery of surrender can be described at all, is to paint a portrait of what it is not. The following, then, is my short list of what surrender is not. Please keep in mind that this list is anything but exhaustive.

1. *Surrender is not passivity.* Passivity is most often, if not always, unhealthy, and surrender has far more to do with patience than with any behavior even approaching a subtle form of psychopathology. Passivity owns no faith and is guided only by fear. And let's face it, fear is the absolute worst, and most dangerous, emotional predicate upon which to base any decision we can ever be called upon to make.

Passivity means avoidance and denial and is often undergirded by the self-imposed conviction that one is incapacitated. When I believe that I "can't" and I get stuck in the "can'ts," then I am being passive.

Step 1 is an admission of "can't," but if we stop there, we will fall into a passive emotional/behavioral vortex quicker than a grub can turn into a June bug. Step 3 is the way out of passivity. It is truer than rain in April that I may be powerless over a good bit of my life, but it is equally true that there is one who is not powerless. Through Step 3 and through the act of surrender, I willingly plug into that power, and I am no longer passive.

2. *Surrender is not agitation.* Agitation by my definition is the expenditure of energy on anything that does not touch the problem. I once was acquainted with a pastoral staff of a large church in a northern state that sought to solve one particular problem through the process of agitation. The problem was that the organist, who was a gifted, retired professor of sacred music, had grown so feeble and so racked with the pain caused by arthritis in his fingers that he could no longer effectively play the hymns or accompany the anthems the choir sang.

Instead of anyone's confronting the problem head-on, for close to a decade the church suffered in the painful presence of the man's slowly deteriorating condition. Committee meetings were held, anonymous letters were even written by members of the congregation to the organist himself, but no one ever bothered to confront the situation with the obvious truth.

For years the man played on, and the entire congregation suffered. Finally the old man succumbed to heart disease and toppled over in the middle of his favorite Saturday afternoon opera broadcast.

The problem was solved, but not without years of agony undergirded by a solid and, I might add, sick commitment to systemic avoidance. Such is agitation, and agitation is the antithesis of Step 3.

3. *Surrender is not a superficial religious ritual.* In fact, I am not certain that surrender has much at all to do with religion. No, as I reflect on my own process of daily surrender, the more I come to see religion as the institutional expression of faith. I view surrender quite differently. I see it as an individual, personal, and, therefore, noninstitutional relationship with God.

Surrender cannot be predicted, scripted, or institutionalized. The best metaphor I have for it concerns my annual trips to Big Bend National Park where I float in a raft through the magnificent Santa Elena Canyon. When I step into the raft, I surrender. There is no fanfare. No candles are lit, no pipe organ pumps out a hymn, and no recitation of pious verbiage is lifted to the desert sky. I simply make a commitment to a journey and, in that process, I permit the river to be my guide. In a very real sense I surrender to its "wisdom."

Consistently, the river has proven to be a wonderful, trustworthy guide. It carries me over rapids and through deep canyons and delivers me, on occasion, to whitewater torrents. Once I have begun the journey in this

Step 3: I turn my life over to God.

desolate land, there is absolutely no turning back. It is virtually impossible to hike out of this remote desert canyon; therefore, wisdom requires that I permit the river to remain in charge of my destiny.

I am not at all passive on this journey in that I assist the river in guiding me through the safest "gates" so that I, along with my fellow sojourners, will not be sucked beneath the surface by some invisible, but still-powerful, hydraulic force. In a very real sense, I cooperate with the river, but the cardinal principle of river travel is this: never, and by this I mean NEVER fight the river. The professional guides on the Rio Grande term such a foolish effort "pushing the river." It is an invariably fruitless exercise to attempt to push any river. Consequently, the only wise choice is to cooperate completely with it and surrender fully to its wisdom.

The same is true with God. We are called to surrender to a will and to an intelligence that is much higher than anything you and I can possibly imagine from our anthropocentric frame of reference, to borrow again from Matthew Fox. I am convinced that, if we are willing to surrender and demonstrate our faith one day at a time by cooperating with God as opposed to "pushing the river," we will, in time, discover the following amazing truth: what God has in mind for us is far better than anything that we could have conceived for ourselves.

I know this will sound to many readers like one more preacher's pie in the sky, but I believe it to be true in that I have experienced its veracity dramatically in my own life.

Only a year prior to my writing this book, I was literally desperate to know what God would have me do with this life and with what I perceived to be my call to ministry. Daily I walked the streets and byways contiguous to the University of Texas, praying silently, but earnestly, for any kind of sign, symbol, guidance, or insight.

At one institution, where in my own subjective impression I thought that I might make a significant contribution, I did not even make the short list for an open position. Following that particular disappointment, I applied at two churches where I knew there to be openings on the pastoral staff, and both churches said in effect, "Thank you, but we're not interested."

Then something very surprising, even startling, occurred. I was invited to resign from my job. I had never actually been let go before, but I was dismissed one Thursday morning. To this day I don't really understand the machinations, both conscious and unconscious, of that painful incident, but the bottom line was that I was turned out, let go, and abandoned.

Immediately following the notice of my dismissal, and with no opportunity to mount any kind of defense with people whom I had come to regard as my friends, I honestly did not know what else to do but to walk. Stunned by the news, I slowly lifted myself from the stuffed chair in my office. I shuffled outside into the beautiful courtyard of the century-old church, and I stared into the cold February sky and uttered only two words: "I surrender!" That was it. Those two words were all that I knew to mumble. "I surrender!" I whispered a second time.

Four days later I was invited to join the staff as a resident teacher, writer, and pastoral counselor of the most dynamic, exciting church I have ever even heard about. As of this writing, I have been on the pastoral staff of Riverbend Church one full year, and I can say without even the slightest exaggeration that this has been the most rewarding, fulfilling, and meaningful year of my life.

There are days when I do ask myself this question: "What am I doing on the staff of a Baptist church when I am ordained in the Presbyterian Church?" My answer always comes back to my moment of agony beneath the live oak trees in the courtyard of another church where the year before, I was dismissed. I am here, today, doing my work and loving it because I believe that this is where God would have me be.

I sometimes think of writing the good man (and he is a good man) who terminated me so that I might offer my sincere thanks to him, but I suspect that he would perceive any such response from me as sick sarcasm. Therefore, I refrain from it. But in truth, I am grateful to the man for shoving my back against the proverbial wall and compelling me to do what I had put off doing for years—surrendering.

Suffice it to say, then, that surrender is not some intellectual head trip. No, surrender is so much more. In truth, it is an excruciatingly painful shift in the foundation stones of our very character. When I was a kid, I once tumbled off of the back end of a go-cart and fractured one of the bones in my right arm. For a time the immediate pain was close to unbearable, but I have discovered that the emotional, psychic pain of my own experience with surrender to be even more intense.

4. Finally, *surrender is not the expansion of the ego.* It is not some vain exercise in the building of self-esteem. No, in fact, it is just the opposite. It is the development of the ego for a single purpose—so that we might give it away to God and to other human beings. It is the giving away of the sum total of my struggles to become a functioning, competent adult through the offering to a power much higher than myself these words: "Here, this life is yours. Do with it as you wish. It is entirely yours. From this day forward, one day at a time, I will cooperate with you. Of course, and let's get this straight between us at the git-go, I will make all manner

Step 3: I turn my life over to God.

of mistakes in the context of my surrendering. There will be times when I will yank my ego out of your hands. But just for today, I invite you to be in charge."

The final question is, of course, How? How do we surrender? I hope those of you who read this book will not be placed in a position of being shoved against the wall, though I suspect that many of you have both been there and can identify fully with the fear that gripped me in that awkward, terrifying, wonderful, blessed moment a year ago.

My recommendation is that you surrender a little bit of your life every day. Begin with the small things. In time you will be ready to give up the bigger, more precious parts of your self. With patience and practice, you will be ready to give it all to God.

Begin with surrendering what you obviously cannot control. Surrender such issues as worry, guilt, small fears, irrational thoughts, and the need to control a loved one. Do not attempt to surrender these issues for all time. Simply make your prayer something like this: "Today, *and just for today*, I will surrender my need to control my child. I will give up *just for today* worrying about whether or not Cousin Harry ever gets his life together. Today, *and just for today*, I will pray for God's will to be done in the context of Aunt Bertha's cancer, but then I will give the cancer and Aunt Bertha to God. And I will get on with my day, be peaceful and centered in all that it could possibly mean to trust God."

Try this exercise, and make it your discipline for two full weeks. Keep a daily journal, and I predict that at the end of fourteen days you will discover that you have far more peace than you have experienced in years, perhaps even in your entire life.

Surrender, like anything else, requires discipline, and discipline means practice. Where there is any kind of efficacious practice, there must also, of course, be a strong commitment to patience.

I wish to conclude this chapter on Step 3 by sharing a story that both demonstrates the power of patience and serves as my own model for all that it could possibly mean to be patient with someone else or with myself.

Janet, a special education teacher, was also a member of the church I served for a decade in Dallas. Most every Sunday she would stop by my station at the church sanctuary door and invite me to visit her classroom at my convenience.

I am not certain why I consistently eschewed her invitations except for the fact that I have never been particularly comfortable, for whatever reason, in the presence of mentally retarded children. I have worked successfully, and quite comfortably, as a pastoral counselor with mentally retarded adults on numerous occasions, but there is something about being with such children that stirs a deep, inexpressible pain in me.

I resisted Janet's persistence until I could locate no further excuses to toss at her. Finally, one warm, spring day just before the school semester slipped into summer, I visited Janet's classroom. Nothing could have prepared me for what I was to witness. Her class consisted of only three children. All of them were severely brain damaged.

Her learning objective for one little girl, Treva, was simply to teach her to hold a fork and to raise the thing to her mouth. That had been the single objective for the entire year.

I watched in fascination as Janet worked diligently with Treva. From my place at the door I counted each time I heard the fork hit and then rattle atop the table of Treva's high chair. Forty-one. Forty-two. Forty-three, I counted. At somewhere in the high fifties, Janet stopped, arose from her small seat adjacent to Treva's high chair, hugged the little girl, and said, "We're gonna make it, Treva. You and me, kid. We're gonna make it."

As I wiped the tears from my eyes, I followed Janet to the teachers' lunchroom, where she had promised we would share a snack. After I regained my composure, I asked the question now burning in my soul. "Why?" (I have since learned, you will recall that "Why?" questions are in the main useless.) My young teacher friend smiled at me and offered three words I have etched permanently on my heart: "Because she matters."

I am convinced God regards us in much the same way that Janet viewed her precious students—with an indescribable sense of patience. Treva drops her eating utensil, but I am just as likely to let fall my clumsy efforts at what it means to surrender. In my own mind, it is helpful to remember Janet's amazing patience. I fully believe that God is even more patient with you and me than Janet was with Treva.

Step 3 is, as I've said, to me the most difficult of the 12. Please don't get discouraged if you don't accomplish it at first. Few, I suspect, have. A man I hardly know had to shove my back against the wall before I could finally utter those two wonderful, healing, terrifying words: "I surrender!"

The New Testament teaches us that many are called but few are chosen. What does that mean? Perhaps it has something to do with the fact that, while all of us are called to surrender, few of us really ever do. I am not certain of this interpretation, of course, but I do know this: surrender is difficult; it requires enormous courage. The fact is that all of us are called to surrender, but few of us ever really do.

Step 3: I turn my life over to God.

The fact remains that inner peace requires the courage to trust that which transcends all five of our senses. As the title of this book suggests, it sounds simple, but this Step is difficult, very difficult.

Therefore, be patient, and even kind, with yourself in working this Step. In the program we often say, "Easy does it." To that I would add, "And may God bless you with courage."

References

[1] Viktor E. Frankl, *The Unconscious God*, reprint (New York: Simon and Shuster, 1975), p. 16.
[2] Ibid., p. 22.
[3] Ibid.
[4] Ibid.
[5] Ibid., p. 23.
[6] Ibid., p. 31.
[7] Ibid.
[8] Ibid., p. 27.
[9] Ibid., p. 35.
[10] Ibid., p. 55.
[11] Ibid., p. 54.
[12] Ibid., p. 57.
[13] Thomas Merton, *The Sign of Jonas* (New York: Harcourt Brace Jovanovich, 1953), p. 112.
[14] Ibid.
[15] Gerald May, pp. 92–94.
[16] Thomas Merton, *New Seeds of Contemplation*, p. 104.
[17] Gerald May, p. 138.
[18] Thomas Merton, *New Seeds of Contemplation*, p. 159.
[19] Ibid.

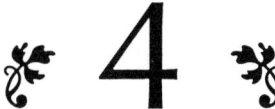

Whatever you have said in the dark shall be heard in the light, and what you have whispered in private rooms shall be proclaimed upon the housetop.

Luke 12:3 RSV

Step 4: *I make a fearless moral inventory of myself.*

Step 4 is the courageous step of contemplation and action that intentionally shepherds us toward the difficult integration of our pseudoselves (false selves) with the authentic self, or who we really are. When this integration begins, we take an important, even crucial, step on the meandering path toward wholeness.

Let's get something straight from the start regarding this step. This 4th Step is *not* an occasion for shame. Shame means to feel bad about who you are. The experiencing of some guilt is, of course, necessary and, in fact, even good for us. This kind of healthy guilt is best termed "remorse," but it would be a mistake, and quite counterproductive to healing, for us to get stuck in some kind of "shame cycle" where we feel overcome by remorse, neurotic guilt, or shame.

I invite you to be grateful for your guilt. Its presence in your life is also a gift of grace. It quite simply means that you are not a sociopath. It also conveys the truth that you are, deep-down, a very healthy individual.

But to hang onto guilt is about as fruitless as going fishing without a hook; it produces absolutely nothing. God is not in favor of it, in that hanging onto our guilt does nothing to promote the kingdom; it serves only to make us sick.

Parenthetically, there are essentially two types of guilt. The first is neurotic guilt: anger at the ego, or the self, for something for which we are not responsible. A person who suffers from this kind of guilt most likely stands in need of some serious therapeutic work on what, in counseling terminology, are known as ego boundaries. To feel guilty or angry at yourself for something for which you have (or had) no responsibility is counter to growth and, quite frankly, also antithetical to the kingdom of God.

I love my daughter more than words can describe. As I write this book, she is, thank God, progressing quite well in her young life and, since the day of her birth more than two decades ago, she has been, and remains, the delight of her parents' lives. But let us imagine, simply for the sake of illustration, that one day she decided to throw her life away by getting hooked on crack cocaine. Further, let us imagine that she began to deal the deadly poison and was arrested and sent to waste decades of her precious life in some prison cell.

If such a tragic scenario were to occur, I would hurt so badly that I know of no adjectives that could adequately describe the pain. There can be absolutely no doubt that her mother and I would venture through our own dark nights of the soul in a way, I suspect, that we had never been called upon before to experience.

But let's be clear about one thing: her decision to wreck her life would *not* be my decision, neither would it be her mother's, or anyone else's. If I were healthy, I would stop myself from embracing any real guilt in the wake of her self-imposed tragedy. For, you see, the choice for addiction lies *always* in the heart and in the mind of the individual who makes such a tragic choice. Of course, in the wake of this tragedy I might ask my friends, and even God, "Where did we go wrong?" But such a question is nothing more than the expression of what is termed "neurotic guilt."

Whether or not she chooses to worship at the throne of the false god we know as addiction, the fact is that I went wrong many places in my daily participation in the task of rearing my daughter. I certainly made my share of mistakes with her. There can be no real question about that. At times, I, no doubt, indulged her far too much with attention, concern, and, most of all, things. At other times, my disease, which manifested itself in her childhood by my compulsion for work, caused me to withdraw from her and deny her needs. However, even though I was a far less than perfect father, any decision she might make to displace God for an addiction to crack cocaine would always be *her* decision, and *not* mine

Step 4: I make a fearless moral inventory.

for her. (Because her mother will read this book, I wish to reiterate that our daughter is a lovely, bright, intelligent college student on her way to making some kind of significant contribution in the world. *Fortunately, she has not chosen to addict herself to crack cocaine or any other illicit drug.*)

Again, then, neurotic guilt is to feel anger and to express anger at oneself in the wake of some disappointment that occurs beyond the boundaries of one's control. Healthy guilt is what I term "remorse." Remorse is an appropriate feeling and can serve effectively as a healing force in our lives. Remorse, or healthy guilt, is what I feel when I am angry at myself for messing up, or for being a boor, which is the one place in my life where I can be "perfect." Remorse, then, is what I normally feel in the wake of awareness of my own sin.

The good, in fact, the wonderful, news is that both neurotic guilt and genuine remorse are quite treatable through the miracle of these 12 Steps. I offer this information because many, many people have worked the first three Steps only to get snagged by their own overwhelming sense of guilt once they hit Step 4.

As I mentioned at the outset of this chapter, Step 4 involves discovering and *then* embracing our authentic selves vis-à-vis the inauthentic or what is termed the "pseudo-self." In a very real sense, this process delivers us from the pseudo-self of our adaptations to the culture that reared us to the authentic, real self of God's creation.

My belief about making the moral inventory is that this is the best way, in fact, the only way I know, that we can begin a disciplined process toward what it means to be a whole person. To move toward wholeness, we must first come to grips with how it is that we keep ourselves from such growth through our insistence upon being inauthentic, or false, in our relationship with God, with our neighbors, and with ourselves. This awareness of our inauthentic self must necessarily precede any venture down the path that leads to the discovery of the authentic self.

One promise I will make (and you will notice that I have not made many promises in this book) is this: if you persevere with Step 4 *(and that is a prodigious IF!)*, you will eventually begin to like and then even to love who you are. No matter what you've done or what you have failed to do, you will end up loving yourself.

Why? (There is that question again.) I can make this bold assertion only because the truth of who we are as well as who we are called to be lies in the Scripture. The Word of God proclaims to those who have the will to hear it that you and I were created in the image of the divine. Therefore, when we dare to launch into any process of self-discovery, we will inevitably end up discovering God as well.

We cannot expect to arrive immediately or easily at the recognition of our creation in God's image, but with effort, courage, and perseverance, we will, in time, discover that the *authentic* self, as opposed to the pseudo-self, is *always*, without exception, friendly and, ultimately, loving simply because the authentic self is joined inextricably to the one who made us in the image of all that it could possibly mean to love.

But this probing process into the discovery of the authentic self is *never* easy. Therefore, I recommend that you do this Step with a trusted friend who has gone there before you, so to speak. This means do the Step with an adult who has safely accomplished *and* completed the Step. Do not, repeat, DO NOT attempt this Step with someone who has not completed Step 4 safely. That would be tantamount to visiting a therapist who has never been in serious treatment for his or her own demons.

Also, in working Step 4, keep in mind that our personalities are very, very complex. John Sanford paints as good a picture of the complexity of the human personality as anyone I have ever read: "The personality is every bit as varied and complex as the body. If a portion of our true nature is denied, we suffer throughout. We cannot afford to exclude anything that belongs to us, for whatever we have denied suffers and this suffering is a part of the body of the whole."[1]

Once again, I fully believe that Step 4 is about wholeness, or, in Sanford's words, healing the suffering that occurs when any part of us is "denied." Without this Step, any serious movement toward wholeness is, in my view, virtually impossible. Further, I have come to recognize in the context of my own recovery that wholeness is now my vocation. Only a few years ago, I would have worked hard to convince you, assuming your interest, of course, that my vocation was ministry. Vocation, according to my former definition, meant proclaiming the Word. It also involved teaching about the great theologians and offering efficacious counsel from the perspective of what the Scripture terms a "listening heart." Vocation also meant to write books, articles, and my newspaper column.

Today, however, I view the term "vocation" quite differently. Through my recovery, I have come to believe that my avocation is ministry (another avocation is fishing!) while my *true* vocation is now, and has been all along, wholeness. C. G. Jung termed this movement I have experienced in my own life toward wholeness the process of "individuation."[2] He firmly believed that this movement toward what it meant to become an authentic individual was the source of all true health. The more I practice the principles of the 12 Steps, the more I discover myself identifying with Jung's insistence upon individuation's being central to what it

Step 4: I make a fearless moral inventory.

means to be a healthy, whole human being. This is why I have come to believe that, without first working a solid Step 4, there can be no real beginning of this process. And without any significant movement toward wholeness, we will never, of course, come to know inner peace.

Saint Gregory of Nyssa tells us, "The soul who is troubled is near unto God."[3] How can this be, we want to ask, and how does this notion line up with what Jung has taught us about individuation? My conclusion is that both statements line up straighter than new-strung barbed wire. You see, the process of individuation is a difficult, at times even excruciatingly painful, process that is invariably supported by God and that employs mystical love in a manner that is, of course, difficult for us to comprehend. I view God as involved in the process in this way: God loves us so much that God intentionally stirs us up with pain and symbols (symptoms) until we finally begin the process of returning to who God intended us to be, or to the authentic self, or to a strong sense of our own individuation. Unless we make that return to "authenticity" and wholeness, the symbols not only continue, but increase in intensity.

In my days of street ministry I knew an intelligent, very sensitive young African American named Robert. I recall two terribly poignant scenes that I shared with him. The first was far less dramatic than the second.

In the first episode, I recall pushing open the outside door to the church sanctuary immediately following a wedding I had performed only to discover Robert cowering in a shadowy corner as he injected a needle full of heroin into a bloated vein. I left him to his misery on that dark night without uttering a word to this suffering man, and, feeling more than a little embarrassed, I ushered the wedding party and assembled family and guests out a different door. Months later, I arrived at the downtown church early one rainy Sunday morning to discover the building literally surrounded by police cars. Chaos reigned. I identified myself to an officer who had blocked an intersection with his vehicle, and I quickly parked my car in the church parking garage. I walked to the sanctuary side of the building and, much to my shock, I discovered Robert once again, this time gasping for breath as he lay clinging to the narrow trunk of a ligustrum.

He had been shot by an unknown assailant who was now on the run from the police. As he breathed his last, I heard him whisper: "God. God. God."

For as long as the Lord gives me to live on this earth, I will *never* forget that tragic scene, neither will I let go of those three poignant, wrenching, heart-stopping words. "God. God. God," he whispered, and then he died.

In my estimation, Robert was both consciously, and at the same time, unconsciously attempting to make it home before he actually arrived there. In the process of dying, his path and destination suddenly became one and the same, and in his final minute and with his last breath, he recognized the intersection of the two in one compelling, unforgettable word: God.

This man had invested a lifetime in avoiding the anxiety that invariably attends the process of individuation. In the process of his adamant insistence upon avoidance, he lived with such internal, unconscious terror that he daily numbed his pain with cheap wine and whatever illicit drugs he could muster the resources to purchase on the street. In a very real sense, he wasted (in my judgment) his life, prior to his tragic death in a Presbyterian flowerbed, by swapping one kind of anxiety for another.

Theologian Paul Tillich describes powerfully the inescapable anxiety that comes with "being" in this existence we call life:

Man's being is not only given to him, but also demanded of him. He is responsible for it, literally, he is required to answer, if he is asked, what he has made of himself. He who asks him is his judge, namely he himself. The situation produces anxiety which in relative terms is the anxiety of guilt and in absolute terms, the anxiety of self-rejection or condemnation. Man is asked to make of himself what he is supposed to become, to fulfill his destiny. In every act of moral, self-affirmation man contributes to the fulfillment of his destiny, to the actualization of what he potentially is.[4]

I know of no better way to ground myself in what I believe Step 4 is truly about than to embrace Tillich's words. There can be no real argument here. Step 4 generates anxiety more quickly than gossip travels through a small town. But the fundamental, and perhaps even ironic, point that I sense Tillich is hammering home here is this: whether or not we choose to take Step 4 in the effort of moving toward the authentic self, we will, in truth, always remain anxious.

We are given an interesting choice, it seems. We can remain stuck in the inauthentic self and remain forever anxious, *or* we can courageously decide to discover the authentic self and then feel anxious. One anxiety leads to certain misery and, I suspect, the eventual death of the spirit, if not of life itself; the second kind of anxiety serves as a guide, if you will, that leads us ultimately to the destiny that God has planned for us. With either decision, however, we will be anxious.

The more we avoid questioning ourselves, the more anxious we inevitably become. The more we put off taking a hard look at our destiny, which once more I truly believe my dying friend Robert was doing with his last utterance, the more tense, confused, and chaotic our lives be-

Step 4: I make a fearless moral inventory.

come. If I have learned anything at all in this program of recovery, it is the simple truth that the only way out of anything, including this existential anxiety of which Tillich writes so eloquently or the dread that invariably attends any honest evaluation of my life, is to plow straight through it.

It is not, therefore, the purpose of Step 4 to shame ourselves or to bury our egos beneath layer upon layer of neurotic guilt. No, I am absolutely convinced, after having accomplished this Step for myself, that Step 4's true purpose is to place us on a path on which, in time, we will experience what perhaps will be a dramatic rendezvous with destiny, if I might borrow from Franklin D. Roosevelt. But keep in mind, this rendezvous has nothing to do with political hyperbole; rather, it is grounded in the truth of our need to discover where it is God would have us go and, even more important, who it is God would have us become.

A big part of working Step 4 involves the willingness to face our fears. If I am willing to do that, I am on my way to reducing the anxiety in that I have stepped in the certain direction of that which is true for my life. One of the greatest fears that may likely come to visit us in the process of working this Step is the fear that defends against the uncovering, if you will, of what is termed "repression" by mental health professionals.

Repression is an ego defense that makes the conscious unconscious. It is a psychological trick of sorts, in that it prevents me from knowing what it is that I need to know simply because my mind, in its own primitive way, is attempting to take care of me or, more accurately, to protect me from information and experiences that it believes I am not yet emotionally equipped to handle. The fact is that I must investigate this psychological trick, or repression, if I ever hope to become conscious. And I cannot fully work Step 4 and remain unconscious or repressed.

Repression in a very real sense restricts growth. Otto Rank describes the impact of any such restriction upon our continued growth. When we restrict ourselves in any significant way, "we feel ourselves guilty on account of the unused life, the unlived life."[5] Rollo May further suggests that the concept of "repression may be understood from the perspective of one's relationship to one's own potential, that is the concept of the unconscious should be enlarged to include the individual's repressed potential."[6]

After ingesting these two insights, we must, I believe, once again pose the question of the role of repression in our own process of integration: What role does repression play in preventing us from fully potentiating our authentic self? Rollo May asks this question in a far more articulate manner than I ever could:

> *What goes on that he [man] chooses or is forced to choose, to block off from his awareness of something that he knows and on another level something that knows that he knows.... The unconscious, then, is not to be thought of as a reservoir of impulses, thoughts, and wishes that are culturally unacceptable. I define it rather as those potentialities for knowing and experiencing that the individual cannot or will not actualize.*[7]

The concept that each individual has unique potential that yearns to be realized goes back to the ancient Greeks. It has also long been my view that such a concept is evidenced in the New Testament in Jesus' transactions with ordinary people. In my mind, this is exactly what transpired in the story of Zacchaeus (Luke 19: 1f.), the miserly tax collector and professional cheat who experienced some kind of mysterious transformation that delivered him to a new experience with generosity. Such generosity, I suspect, was the manifestation of his recognition and the bringing to full fruition of the "authentic self" that Jesus saw in him.

I remain convinced that the discovery and uncovering of our individual potential is the primary, though certainly not the sole, purpose of our working Step 4. This Step is one, though certainly not the only, path to the unconscious. Somewhere in our lives, we have learned to or, at some level, perhaps, decided to repress our potential in that we have buried beneath layers of "unawareness" the truth, *along with other bits of information,* of who we have been created to be. Step 4, done correctly, with healthy emotional support, and gently and slowly, can probe effectively into and even through a lifetime's worth of repression.

The point is this: there can be no serious move toward wholeness and integration until we do some very serious and skillful archaeological work into our own personalities around the salient issue of how it is we have stopped ourselves from bringing to *full* fruition the gifts God has bestowed so generously upon us. This gentle digging I term very simply Step 4.

I view Step 4, then, as the primary opportunity in our recovery to make the unconscious conscious, to recognize, one day at a time, the exact nature as well as the machinations of our archaic defense mechanisms, and to plot carefully and intentionally a new course toward both God and who it is God made us to be.

I find it fascinating that, while the fourth cardinal sin is sloth (which in my mind is the sin of failing to do with one's life all that one knows that one can do), in a very real sense, it is precisely the 4th Step of recovery that is designed, I believe, to shepherd us one Step at a time beyond our sick attachment to sloth. (Another, and perhaps more modern, way of describing sloth is to view it in the more clinical terms of avoidance and

Step 4: I make a fearless moral inventory.

passivity.)

If all of us were allowed to grow up in nurturing, loving environments where there was no abuse and where we were encouraged to bring to fruition the gifts God has given us, there would be no need whatsoever for Step 4 in that there would be no need for serious repression or any kind of emotional restriction. But, of course, this is anything but a perfect world. Once, when I was a kid sitting in the half-empty Cotton Bowl following a particularly difficult defeat by a team well acquainted with losing, I happened to offer a brief commentary on the game to an older gentleman seated next to me who apparently shared my disappointment. I said innocently enough, more to myself than to him, "If we had not fumbled in the fourth quarter, we would have won." He stood, dusted the popcorn from his tweed trousers, looked toward heaven, and said, "Kid, if a bullfrog had wings he wouldn't bump his butt every time he hopped."

Those words were not the most profound commentary on life that I would ever hear, but I've never forgotten them. We live in a world where "if" really doesn't matter. The truth is that most of us did not have our needs sufficiently met in childhood.

I was far more fortunate than most in that I cannot conceive of being reared in a more nurturing or loving family, but the vast majority of the people I see daily in my role as a pastoral counselor cannot make the same claim. For them, the environment in which they were reared simply did not encourage them to be who God made them to become.

Karen Horney writes about the importance of a caring context in which the realization of each child's full potential is actively encouraged. According to her, under favorable conditions a human being will naturally develop an intrinsic potential just as a seed will develop into a healthy plant. In her view, psychopathology develops when adverse conditions conspire to inhibit a child from growing toward the full realization of his or her natural possibilities. The damage is accomplished when the child loses sight of his or her potential and develops another self-image, an "idealized self" toward which the child directs life energies. The consequence of this is that the child pays a prodigious price by maintaining that alienation from the self that invariably occurs. The discrepancy between authentic potential and the idealized self generates contempt that the individual must endure throughout life.[8]

Abraham Maslow says much the same thing about the denial of one's potential:

If the essential core of the person is denied or suppressed, he gets sick, sometimes in obvious ways sometimes in subtle ways... This inner core is delicate and subtle and easily overcome by habit and cultural pressure... Even though denied, it persists underground, forever pressing for actualization. . . . Every falling away from our core, every crime against our nature records itself in our unconscious and makes us despise ourselves.[9]

I wish to reiterate here that it is *not* the purpose of Step 4 to shame us or harangue us with our many shortcomings; rather, its purpose is to provide us with the opportunity for a deep, and rigorous, evaluation that puts us once again in touch with the authentic self that is inevitably lost in childhood, where full potentiation of the self was not supported. The purpose of Step 4 is to heal the gulf between who one sees oneself to be and who God made us to be.

Working Step 4 may feel at first like an exercise in self-contempt, but nothing could be farther from the truth. In reality, it is the healing of the self-contempt that is bred, according to Dr. Horney, by a lifetime of alienation from ourselves.

We cannot possibly bridge this gulf overnight. Step 4 must be taken on only with great caution and under the guidance of one who has previously traversed the difficult terrain it presents to us on a daily basis. This is *not* the place to get in a hurry in that it is virtually impossible to integrate the pseudo-self with the best in the authentic self in a matter of days or hours, just as it is impossible to have a broken bone mend at the snap of the fingers. *It simply cannot be done.*

In the simplest way I know how to phrase it, Step 4 is the willing death of the "old self" and it is the birth of something almost entirely new and wonderful. Call it being born again, call it whatever you wish, but please, whatever you do, *don't* rush the process. Like any kind of serious healing, this Step simply cannot be hurried.

Years ago I wrote the following description of a tragic encounter on the streets with a Native American named Jason Three Stars. I include a portion of that piece in this discussion of the repression and the anxiety that occurs in a life when someone is cut off by family or even by a whole culture, which is the case in this story:

On that Monday morning in May, he had mixed 15 hours on a bus with at least two bottles of wine. I thought about apologizing for treaties which were broken more than a century ago. And the truth is that I wanted to whisper to him that the Apache ways are as vulnerable to the city's indifference as a buttercup in a hailstorm.

But I didn't own the opportunity to utter anything comprehensible, because Jason Three Stars was too drunk to stand up, much less to eat a donated bowl of vegetable beef stew. I did touch the crook of his elbow, and he recoiled like a timber rattler. Then he flung a

Step 4: I make a fearless moral inventory.

> Styrofoam cup brimming with milk across a Dallas police officer's shoes.
>
> The officer did what was at the moment necessary. Jason Three Stars, with his smooth cheek pressed against the outside wall of the church, his hands now cuffed, waited for an inhospitable squad car to deliver him to the city justice center.
>
> So I never did have a chance to say anything to him. In a sense, he was gone before he even arrived. I don't know even today what I would have said to him had he given me the chance. But I'll never forget what he said to me between labored breaths with those stainless steel cuffs biting into his pulse, his face pushed against Presbyterian marble. He whispered, "Pastor, I am sorry!"[10]

Another way that I have come to view Step 4 is to see it as the beginning of the spiritual journey. Steps 1 through 3 are the preparation, but, in my view, this is the first Step toward a genuine "homecoming."

Thomas Merton writes, "To say that I am made in the image of God is to say that love is the reason for my existence, for God is love. . . . Love is my true identity. Selflessness is my true self. Love is my true character. Love is my name."[11] Love is our true identity. Merton is absolutely correct. When we come to who God created us to be, or the authentic self, and when we finally decide to "come home to God," we, too, discover that our name all along has been what the monk declared it to be: Love.

My own hunch is that whenever Jesus encountered anyone, he would pose this question silently to himself: "Who could you be if you were not standing in your own way?" The Scripture is filled with stories of people who changed radically after their encounters with Jesus, who mysteriously put them in touch with their authentic sense of self: Levi, the tax collector; a blind beggar named Bartimeaus; and that ornery little runt of a tax collector we know as Zacchaeus hiding in the sycamore tree.

Earlier in this chapter, I quoted several of the great minds of psychology and psychiatry, who framed the anxiety surrounding our lack of integration in fairly clinical language. Quite frankly, I also believe that if we are to be true to the spirit of Step 4, we must also couch our "stuckness" in the inauthentic, or pseudo-self, in theological language.

Simply put, the pseudo-self is another name for sin. As Thomas Merton tells us,

> To say that I was born in sin is to say I came into the world with a false self. I was born in a mask. I came into existence under a sign of contradiction, being someone that I was never intended to be and therefore a denial of what I am supposed to be. And thus I came into existence and nonexistence at the same time because from the very

start I was something that I was not.[12]

I tell people almost daily in my office that I believe that what happened to us in our childhood is not our fault. We were impressionable, defenseless, totally vulnerable human beings back then. But what happened to us in our childhood is today very much our responsibility. And our primary responsibility in this life, as I mentioned at the outset of the discussion of Step 4, is to heed our vocation. Vocation is wholeness, and wholeness, of course, requires the healing of childhood wounds.

God is simultaneously both the shepherd and the destiny of that healing. God is all that we need to heal, but we must first cooperate with God's healing power through the discipline of these 12 Steps.

Sometimes in my own dark moment of the night, when I have experienced some painful slip, I tell myself that there must be more help available than this invisible, mysterious force we know as God. Like any human being, I often long for something, anything, that is tangible, that I can reach out and grab with my tense, trembling fingers.

It is in those dark moments that I am more than a little comforted by the words of the apostle Paul in his second letter to the folks at Corinth (2 Cor. 12:9–10): "My grace is sufficient for you, for my power is made perfect in weakness. I will all the more gladly boast of my weaknesses, that the power of Christ may rest upon me. For the sake of Christ then I am content with weaknesses, insults, hardships, persecutions, and calamities, for when I am weak, then I am strong."

Go back and reread the opening words of that passage. "My grace is sufficient for you." What Paul is telling us, like it or not, is that God's grace is all that we really have. To me, the operative word in this passage is "sufficient." I view this to mean that grace is also all that we could ever possibly need. I know of no better news to offer anyone, including myself, than that one wonderful, terrifying, encompassing word: "sufficient."

I am comforted by these words in my own dark moments, when the authentic self seems as far away as summer did every September of my childhood. "We are afflicted in every way, but not crushed; perplexed, but not driven to despair; persecuted, but not forsaken; struck down, but not destroyed; always carrying in the body the death of Jesus so that the life of Jesus may also be made manifest in our bodies."[13]

Gerald May suggests that essentially we have three choices when it comes to the difficult journey toward wholeness. I offer them in paraphrased form. First, we may deny or avoid God's call by repressing our desire and displacing it with energy. Much of the time we are successful at this, but the call is bound to break through our defenses and haunt us with gentle nudges or hound us with relentless yearnings.

Step 4: I make a fearless moral inventory.

Second, we may reduce the images of spiritual reality into something we believe we can control, as opposed to being dependent upon them.

Finally, we can try to be present to the mystery in a gentle, open-handed way that cooperates with God. This is a simple, courageous attempt to bear as much as one can of reality just as it is. Contemplation is simply trying to face life in a truly undefended and open way.[14]

I've yet to run into a better description of Step 4 than this one. That is exactly what Step 4 is—a willingness to be present to the mystery in a gentle, open-handed way that cooperates with God.

Some years ago I was preaching every Sunday during August at what I suspect could best be described as an "alternative" Presbyterian church. I was honored to preach the Word of God to those good folks beneath a stand of two hundred-year-old live oak trees in a community some twenty miles east of Austin. Never had I been invited to proclaim the Good News in a more resplendent sanctuary. About twelve folks gathered for the Sunday morning worship, including the pastor, who had recently taken a maternity leave from this wonderful, though tiny, congregation of peace-loving, authentic-to-the-core folks.

The pastor's first child was a precious, as well as precocious, two-year-old who was, I thought, aptly named Flannery Grace. She seemed to possess the spunk of the noted short story writer of the same first name, and the child's middle name is, in truth, the name of every child, as well as the name of every human being who is created in the image of God. (Which, of course, is every one of us!)

Following my brief homily, I offered the sacrament to the folks gathered in the shade of the magnificent live oaks. I sensed that Flannery Grace was becoming quite interested in worship now that we were passing around a handsome loaf of homemade bread and a cup of freshly poured grape juice.

As the bread passed by her mother, she paused, tore a chunk of warm bread from the loaf, and handed it to my young friend Flannery Grace. Flannery danced in delight in the shade of the live oaks. She lifted her skirt high above her training pants and then proceeded to pat her rather rotund tummy with her plump little hand. Again she danced, giggled, twirled, and said simply, "Thank you."

I've been serving the bread and the wine to men, women, and children from every walk of life for more than two decades, and never before have I witnessed a more authentic response to a sacramental event than was demonstrated by my young, precocious friend, Flannery Grace.

I have come to regard Step 4 as being like Flannery Grace's response to the sacrament—nothing less than a sacramental event in that, like the bread and the wine, the rigorous and fearless moral inventory invariably carries us to grace. Only grace can answer the riddle of my identity and only grace can deliver me safely to my destination, which all along has been that place, or reality, where I first began. We know that reality as God.

Be careful with yourself in this Step. Remember that there is no corner in God's kingdom where shame is ever appropriate. The apostle is correct: God's grace is sufficient to remove any guilt, even the neurotic kind.

So be gentle in your cooperation with God. Ease into Step 4 as though you were stepping into the refreshing waters of a mountain stream for the first time. Take one step and allow yourself to grow accustomed to both the temperature and the easy flow of the current before you trust enough to lie down so that the mystery of baptism might once again wash away the strong, binding sense of your own sin and restore your soul to wholeness.

Reference

[1] John A. Sanford, *Healing and Wholeness* (New York: Paulist Press, 1977), p. 7.
[2] Ibid., p. 16.
[3] Ibid., p. 8.
[4] Irvin Yalom, *Existential Psychotherapy* (New York: Basic Books, 1980), p. 278.
[5] Ibid.
[6] Ibid.
[7] Ibid.
[8] Ibid.
[9] Ibid. pp. 280.
[10] Bob Lively, *On Earth As It Is . . . Discovering God's Grace in the Ordinary* (Austin: Publication Designers, 1994), pp. 85–87.
[11] Thomas Merton, *New Seeds of Contemplation*, p. 60.
[12] Ibid., pp. 33-34.
[13] 2 Cor. 4: 8–9 RSV.
[14] Gerald May, p. 107.

❦ 5 ❧

Therefore confess your sins to one another, that you may be healed. The prayer of a righteous man has great power in its effects.

James 5:16 RSV

Step 5.   *I admit to God the exact nature of my wrongs.*

Through Step 5, I offer God nothing other than a sincere prayer of confession that lists the *exact* nature of my wrongs, without equivocation, without excuse, without rationalization. What I offer God in this Step is nothing less than the truth, in the best way I know how to articulate it.

But let us also be reasonable with this Step. In fact, and here we must be very careful, the Step does *not* say that I must admit *all* of my wrongs. If I were to attempt such a thing, even if such were possible, I would soon enough find myself so mired in memory and bogged down in details that not even a John Deere tractor with a tow chain could extricate me.

I have decided that the best way to approach this Step is to frame it as a symbol. This concept is in no way intended as any kind of license for prevarication, or what East Texas folks simply call plain old lying. No, if I intend to work this Step, I need to confess all of the wrongs that I can recall. But once again, let us be reasonable. I simply cannot recall them all. The fact is, once I've reached this point in the program, I have discovered that I am such a sinner, in such desperate need of grace, that it is wholly useless for me to pretend otherwise. There are so many sins in my past that about the best I can hope to accomplish is to offer God a slice, or a random sample, if you will, of my own sinful nature.

God knows my nature; there can be no real doubt about that. The point of Step 5 is not to reel off an impressive litany of sins but, rather, to become aware of my nature through the process of carrying one load of poor decisions after another to the throne of grace.

I wrote this book at a marvelous place in the Texas Hill Country known as Mo-Ranch. Twenty years ago, I was leading a summer youth conference in this still-pristine corner of God's kingdom and, on one particularly warm July afternoon, I reclined beneath a large native pecan tree on the banks of the North Fork of the Guadalupe River so that I might write a letter to a trusted friend.

I thought I was alone, but I was surprised to be suddenly covered by a thin shadow. I turned to discover a high school girl approaching me from behind. I sensed immediately that this child was living with some kind of awful misery that I guessed was most likely wholly unnecessary.

She had been a student in the Bible class I was teaching during that week, and yet she had remained so quiet during the course of the several days we shared in this bucolic setting that I scarcely knew even one detail about her, except that her name was "Donna."

She asked if she might sit next to me. I responded with a cheerful, "Certainly."

She nestled so close to me, I found myself feeling strangely uncomfortable. I perceived that she was now physically too close, and I decided that this intrusion upon my personal boundaries could signal only two possibilities: either she was coming on to me sexually (I was about nine years her senior); or, far more likely, she was experiencing deep pain, and her movement toward me was simply her unconscious attempt to discover some kind of solace, which, I suppose, she sensed, or at some level hoped, I might offer.

I decided that the latter possibility was the most likely of the two, and I watched as the tears welling in her eyes rolled down her cheeks.

I chose silence over the offering of any words as I waited for her to speak. Finally she stunned me with this self-definition: "I'm worthless!"

Nothing in my seminary curriculum had prepared me for this moment. I gulped and again decided that now was not the occasion to argue with this child.

She looked at me with eyes clouded in a flood of tears and whispered, "I'm worthless."

What I knew at the time about counseling could have been stored in

Step 5: I admit my wrongs.

my grandmother's thimble with plenty of room remaining for her finger. It was obvious to both of us that I simply did not know how to respond to her pain.

I decided that it was not helpful to engage her in any kind of argument regarding her sense of self, so I asked her this question: "Do you trust me?"

She responded, "Yeah, I guess. I think you're kind of crazy. That's why I like you. You're funny, too. But I had an abortion last year, and my parents don't even know about it. God hates me. I am worthless."

I stood on the banks of the Guadalupe River, tore a river stone from its limestone mooring beneath the green surface of the water, and dropped the thing to the soft mud beyond the boat dock.

She asked, "What's that?"

"Your problem," I answered.

"No, it's just a slimy, dirty, yucky old river rock," she bellowed.

I reminded her: "You said you trusted me."

"Yes," she answered, "I do."

"Pick it up," I ordered, surprising myself that I was being so bold with this child.

She complied and then dropped it as she filled the air with expletives, none of which I have not employed myself when I have found myself just as frustrated as she must have felt at the moment.

Again I admonished her, "Pick it up and follow me."

She did as she was told and followed me as I climbed a steep trail leading to a tall hill above the river canyon where there is located a tall, weathered cross.

Every step of the way that young girl complained, balked, cursed, and fumed. Filled with self-pity, she cried out loud, and then began to scream at me that everyone she had ever heard characterize me was right, after all—I was, indeed, one crazy man.

I chose to remain silent, and when we at long last reached the summit of the hill, I pointed to the wooden cross and said, "Take that ugly, smelly old rock over there and set it at the foot of the cross. Stay there as long as you like. I'll be right here sitting in the shade until you return."

A few years ago, Donna wrote to inform me that she had married an attorney and that they were the proud parents of three precious children.

Without knowing it, Donna worked Step 5, and it is not at all surprising to me that she later experienced healing.

This is also the Step of what I term "accepting responsibility." During my two years in a pastoral counseling residency program, I came to know an amazing young Baptist clergyman named Doyle.

On one particular morning in my memory, Doyle and I and the rest of the residents were gathered to hear a lecture presented by a senior staff counselor. An attractive female member of the staff walked past Doyle's chair and another resident, whom I'll call Homer, and who was seated next to Doyle, whispered a sexist comment regarding the woman's appearance.

Doyle was caught in a weak moment and he snickered out loud. In fact, he snorted. Suddenly a hush fell over the room, and the female faculty member turned abruptly to glare at the place in the room where the laughter had erupted.

Without further provocation, Doyle stood and said something like this: "I abused you just then. I laughed because I am an unhealthy man who is still in the position of seeing women as objects. In that one brief, fleeting moment you were to me nothing more than an object. There is absolutely no excuse for my behavior. I accept full responsibility for any injury that I might have caused you. All that I can do is to confess my sin to you and to God and hope that you will forgive me for being so very insensitive. I do know this. God has forgiven me. Whether or not you forgive me is entirely up to you."

The classroom remained so quiet that I could hear my own heart beating faster than it does when I have just completed a 10K race.

Doyle sat down, and the woman immediately walked to his place and offered him a hug in obvious demonstration of her forgiveness.

Seldom before or since have I been in the presence of one so young who at the same time was so spiritually mature. Spiritual maturity, from my point of view, is predicated upon exactly what my friend did, namely, fully accepting responsibility.

That is also, I suspect, precisely what my young friend Donna did at the foot of the cross. What Step 5 is about is the conscious willingness to face God in the context of prayer with a full-bore commitment to speaking the truth and with a courageous willingness to accept *full* responsibility for how we have sinned.

I have been to college once and to seminary twice, but still I am not sure that I know how to pray. Therefore, I am more than a little comforted by these words from the apostle Paul (Romans 8:26): "Likewise the Spirit helps us in our weakness; for we do not know how to pray as we ought, but the Spirit Himself intercedes for us with sighs too deep for words."

Step 5 is a prayer Step, more specifically, a confessional Step, and the good news is that we don't even have to know how to pray to work it. I am

Step 5: I admit my wrongs.

convinced that God is not at all interested in or impressed by how we pray or by our awkward stabs at elocution. No, I suspect that God is much more interested in one thing about us—sincerity. As Paul reminds us, even when we don't know how to pray for ourselves, the Spirit does the work for us. What more could we ask?

Step 5, then, is about the *full* as opposed to truncated confession of our diluted notions of personal sin. "Sin" is a word that we are not comfortable bantering about in the church today, but, be that as it may, our "sin" is that which must be confessed in this 5th Step if we are to experience any kind of significant healing.

Theologian Paul Tillich describes our difficulty with the word "sin" in his explication of the seventh chapter of Paul's Letter to the Church at Rome:

For I do not do the good I want, but the evil I do not want is what I do. Now if I do what I do not want, it is no longer I that do it, but sin which dwells in me. Tillich continues:

The name of that power is sin. Nothing is more precarious today than the mention of this word among Christians, as well as among non Christians, for in everyone there is a tremendous resistance to it. It is a word that has fallen into disrepute. To some of us it sounds almost ridiculous and is apt to provoke laughter rather than serious consideration. To others, who take it more seriously, it implies an attack on their human dignity. And again, to others—to those who have suffered from it—it means the threatening countenance of the disciplinarian, who forbids them to do what they would like and demands of them what they hate. Therefore, even Christian teachers, including myself, shy away from the use of the word sin. We know how many distorted images it can produce. We try to avoid it, or to substitute another word for it. But it has a strange quality. It always returns. We cannot escape it. It is as insistent as it is ugly. And so it would be more honest—and this I say to myself—to face it and ask what it really is. . . .

It is noteworthy that today, in order to know the meaning of sin, we have to look outside our churches and their average preaching to the artists and writers and ask them. But perhaps there is still another place where we can learn what sin is, and that is our own heart.[1]

What does this have to do with Step 5? Everything. You see, Tillich has nailed our problem. Our problem is not to be found lurking in our "sins"; rather, our problem is simply sin itself. But how do I go to God and say I'm a sinner and have that kind of generic confession make any substantive difference in the way I decide to live this life?

Such confession is nothing more than a vacuous, abstract statement, at best. It's like any kind of recitation that becomes so remote as to disconnect from passionate reality.

When I first joined the staff of Riverbend Church, I recall being somewhat surprised that there was no place in the liturgy for a confession of sin or for any kind of assurance of pardon. At first this "omission" unsettled me a bit. Upon reflection, however, I found myself being glad for the omission in that what I have experienced for a lifetime in the confessional church of my rearing is that we as a church have collectively and, I suspect, unconsciously, reduced the authentic confession of personal sin into the mere recitation of words printed on a church bulletin. And the truth is that I have far more often mumbled those words than I have ever offered them with a deep sense of connection to my own nature. I have come to believe that there is really no place for such a confession of authentic sin in worship, because what we offer in the form of a confession has been so diluted and carefully orchestrated to allow sufficient time for the sermon and the choir's well-rehearsed anthem, that the prayer has long been bereft of any real substance.

Now I know full well that this position will rile my liturgically-minded friends, but then, they've been upset with me for years. So I'll risk it, because I know them to be people of grace.

Step 5 is no mere recitation of high-sounding words having to do with commission and omission; it is that cathartic moment in our lives when we dare to step beyond our façades, when we rip off the masks of our well-worn pretentiousness, and when, for the good of our own souls, we ground ourselves in the truth of what Tillich calls our very nature, which, of course, is sin.

I am convinced that God is not at all interested in the details of our wrongs. No, I suspect that God is far more invested in our healing than in the cataloging of our misdeeds or serious omissions. Further, I have come to believe that any real hope for our healing is invariably predicated upon our being grounded in the truth of our nature. But how can I know my sinful nature without getting in touch with the "evidence"? The evidence of my profound proclivity for sin is contained, of course, in my sins. It is in the process of confessing those very sins that I come to at least a partial awareness of my own sinful nature.

Therefore, when I approach the throne of grace and confess the exact nature of my wrongs, without rationalization or excuse, I experience two realities that make healing possible. First, I get in touch with the fact that the apostle Paul was conveying the truth when he wrote two thousand years ago, "Sin dwells in me." Sin also dwells in my being. It is only

Step 5: I admit my wrongs.

through this act of confession that I finally come to discover sin to be a natural part of my being.

Second, I come to experience the truth of God's grace at a visceral, and even soulful, level. Through this experience, I come to realize, one day at a time, one Step at a time, that God can, through the process of my confession, transform my very nature. God is that powerful! But I will not and I cannot experience the power of God unless I first get in touch with my nature through the process of confession, or what in the program we term working Step 5.

The truth of my nature and the truth of God's power *cannot* be discovered, nor can they possibly be embraced in the abstract. A polite, antiseptic prayer of confession full of all manner of "thees" and "thous" and all kinds of stylish, high-sounding omissions and commissions, does not move me even one step closer to authentic healing. To me, such a prayer is nothing more than a quaint symbol of the truth that God does pardon us; the prayer is far too opaque, and far too disconnected from the reality of my own sinful nature for me to experience any significant healing from its recitation.

It is little wonder to me that the spirituality movement, which has proven itself to be potent enough to usher God's grace into the lives of the broken, has, by necessity, abandoned the institutional church and has again retreated to underground catacombs we in this culture know as church basements. People still worship on Sunday morning in the stained-glass sanctuaries of this culture, but most often, the real healing occurs in the basement, when many of those same pew-sitting folks swap their polite printed confessions for the authentic catharsis regarding their very nature.

While the spirituality movement gains momentum, the traditional institutional church is all too willing, it seems, to have us join in the trivialization of our confessions. Many people have stood before the same altar or chancel for the whole of their lives and confessed their sins every Sunday morning, only to go home and feel just as scared, just as sad, just as angry, and just as unsettled as when they began their day with a donut and cup of fresh-brewed coffee at the beginning of the Sunday school hour. I know this to be true, because before I discovered recovery, this is exactly how I lived my life. I knew that I was supposed to have faith in being healed. The problem was that I didn't know what real faith or authentic healing actually looked like.

If anyone had accused me of hiding from God for all of those years, I would have pronounced them mistaken. After all, I had dedicated most of my life to God, or at least I believed I had. What I discovered in the context of recovery, however, was that, in truth, I had dedicated my existence to the polite, reserved, rather predictable God of the respectable religious organizations of this culture. What I did not realize, however, was that I had displaced God with my beloved institutions.

Institutions are not God. They never have been and they will never be. God is God, and nothing else can ever take God's place. Yes, the truth is that I was hiding from God by obsessing and "compulsing" about God and terming those thoughts and behaviors, at least in my own mind, "obedience." And I avoided God, simply because I was afraid.

Like my two spiritual ancestors, Cain and Jonah, the fact is that for most of my life I, too, hid from God. Why do any of us hide from God? The answer to that is simple. We have learned to be afraid of God. Once again, I rely upon Paul Tillich to provide insight:

The flight from God begins the moment we feel His presence. This feeling is at work in the dark, half conscious regions of our being, unrecognized, but effective; in the restlessness of the child's asking and seeking; of the adolescent's doubts and despairs; of the adult's desires and struggles. God is present, but not as God; He is present as the unknown force in us that makes us restless.

But in some moments He appears as God. The unknown force in us that caused our restlessness becomes manifest as God...Who is our ultimate threat and our ultimate refuge. In such moments it is as though we were arrested in our hidden flight. But it is not an arrest by brute force, but one that has the character of a question. And we remain free to continue our flight. This is what happened to the disciples: they were powerfully arrested when Jesus first called them, but they remained free to flee again. As they did when the moment of trial arrived.[2]

My truth is that I hid from God and still do, simply because I am afraid, I suspect, to embrace my own sinful nature in God's presence. No, I would much rather pretend some other "reality." My experience with such pretentiousness is what Tillich describes when he points out that "the flight from God begins the moment we feel His presence."

I learned the following truth about myself in this discipline of working Step 5: I flee because I simply do not want to accept responsibility. I run from God because I am ashamed, and I hide from God because I am afraid. I recognize full well that I am not alone in the terrible discomfort that attends the acceptance of responsibility, but having company in this kind of misery is wholly irrelevant to my healing. No one can and no one must accept responsibility for my sin but me.

Scott Peck has coined what I believe is a helpful term for our corporate

Step 5: I admit my wrongs.

refusal to accept responsibility. He terms it a "militant ignorance."[3] Militant ignorance, or the avoidance of responsibility, or the fleeing from the presence of holiness, or hiding from God, or whatever you wish to call the attitude and its attendant sick behaviors, is still what ails us and remains a formidable impediment to our healing. To me, militant ignorance and our individual or collective refusal to accept responsibility are exactly the same thing.

Scott Peck holds up that tragic national debacle known as the Vietnam War as a classic example of this culture's collective unwillingness to accept responsibility:

The Vietnam war is one of the best examples I know of this militant ignorance on a grand scale. When the evidence first began to accumulate in 1963 or 1964 that our policies in Indochina weren't working, our first response was to deny that anything was wrong. We said we just needed a couple of more million dollars and a few more special forces. But then the evidence continued to accumulate—our policies clearly weren't working. So what happened then? We sent in more troops, the body count began to escalate, and incidents of brutality became commonplace. It was the time of My Lai. Then as the evidence continued to pour in, we continued to ignore it. Instead, we bombed Cambodia and started talking about peace with honor.

Even today, despite all that we know, some Americans continue to think that we succeeded in bargaining our way out of Vietnam. We didn't bargain our way out of Vietnam—we were defeated. But somehow many still refuse to see this.[4]

Sometimes I wonder what this world would be like if we the people of this nation were to approach the nation of Vietnam and formally apologize, admit that we were wrong, and offer to make sacrificial reparations for war crimes against their civilization. And what would happen if we the people were to work a collective Step 5 and admit in some manner of harmonious corporate expression that what we did to Native Americans was then and remains in many respects criminal?

What would this nation be like if we the Anglo people of this culture apologized to those of African lineage for hauling their ancestors to this continent shackled in some slave ship? I've been alive close to half a century now, and never have I heard or experienced one such corporate apology.

The sad fact is, you and I probably never will experience such a thing in our lives. Any politician who would mount a campaign for the expression our corporate responsibility for crimes committed in the name of whatever national policy was in place at the moment would never be elected. If she were elected, she could never remain in office with an attitude that even hints that we the people should accept responsibility for even one of our collective sins.

Obviously, the culture opposes such acceptance, and even the institutional church has trivialized the very passionate act of confession and reduced the opportunity for catharsis to an innocuous relic wedged somewhere between the opening hymn and reading of the Scripture.

I don't invest very much energy worrying about such grandiose matters these days. Step 5 calls *me* to accept responsibility by admitting to God the exact nature of *my* wrongs. If I do that, I eventually come to know myself as well as my nature, and I also come to experience the truth of God's amazing power to heal me. I can't make anyone else take Step 5, and even if I possessed such power, I would not use it because I would no doubt misuse it and sin even more against one of my brothers or sisters.

God grants us all manner of freedom. That is the hallmark, I believe, of God's love for us. Faith is always our choice. We can work Step 5 or we can ignore it and trick ourselves into believing that we don't need to confess the exact nature of our wrongs. But whatever our decision, we are always free to choose healing or to remain stuck in a deep pool of denial, like some catfish dropped in a well.

Robert Bly believes that the United States has achieved the first culture of systemic denial in the modern world. The following are his reflections on the matter:

The health of any nation's soul depends on the capacity of adults to face the harsh facts of the time. But the covering up of painful emotions inside us and the blocking out of the fearful images coming from outside have become in our country the national and private style. We have established, with awesome verve, the animal of denial as the guiding beast of the nation's life. The inner city collapses, and we build bad housing projects rather than face bad education, lack of jobs, and persistent anger at black people. When the homeless increase, we build dangerous shelters rather than face the continuing decline in actual wages. Of course we know this beast lives in every country; we have been forced lately to look at our beast.[5]

Denial places us in what I term an "existential purgatory," where we are neither alive nor dead. When I served as associate pastor on the staff of the First Presbyterian Church in Dallas, I was the daily witness to an obvious purgatory. I saw it in the faces of the men and women who had been defeated by life and who, for whatever complex set of reasons, found themselves homeless in Dallas, Texas.

Step 5: I admit my wrongs.

Daily they trudged into the soup kitchen, and as I came to know them, and much later came to love them as brothers and sisters, I began to sense the painful nature of their dilemma. The vast majority of these good folks were afraid—terrified was more like it—of living because they had not made it in this world and this culture had, at best, let them down and, at worst, had abused them terribly. And conversely, I came to understand that they were equally frightened of dying. I saw them as trapped in some kind of cosmic purgatory, or in-between place.

I was once naïve enough to believe that such a dilemma was the province of only the homeless. I have since come to believe, however, that Robert Bly is far more accurate in his description of an entire culture caught in the throes of denial. I, for one, was in denial for decades and growing increasingly comfortable with my pain, daily repressing my disconnection from my authentic self while tossing in God's direction an occasional, well-written prayer of confession.

But Step 5 knocked me out of denial the way a mule kicks an empty milk pail and delivered me, thank God, to the very threshold of my spiritual awakening. I could not possibly have remained in denial and been aware at the same time. Such would be like being in Chicago and Laredo at exactly the same moment. I'm either one place or the other, or on a plane somewhere between the two, but the fact remains that I have to be someplace.

Step 5, if we choose to follow it with sincerity, yanks us out of denial and shepherds us to the throne of grace, where we will likely tremble before a loving God who longs to redeem us.

When I decide to make that confession, it is then that I accept responsibility. Once I have accepted responsibility, I become, perhaps for the first time in my life, aware. Denial, then, becomes nothing more dangerous than a bad memory vibrating in the rearview mirror of my own consciousness.

Why does the 12-Step program work? If there is one answer to that question, it has to be because our humble request for healing is grounded in the absolute truth of our sinful nature. The games are over, the ineffectual defense mechanisms are put away like toys we long ago outgrew, and a lifetime of denial is surrendered to the mysterious, healing power of God's grace.

Scott Peck says "AA [or 12 Steps] works because it is a program of spiritual conversion, teaching people why they must go forward through the desert—namely, toward God."[6]

I wrote that Step 3, or what is termed "surrendering," is for me the most difficult of the 12 Steps. I stand by what I wrote, but I also believe

Simple Steps...Costly Choices

that it is difficult in the "culture of denial," as Robert Bly describes our society, even to admit that we are wrong. I see this difficulty played out daily in my office when I work with couples who are experiencing prodigious pain in their interactions with one another. At some time in their relationship, perhaps many years, even decades, before, they professed to love each other. Today, however, as they sit before me squabbling, it is obvious to me that they would much rather be as far apart as possible, given the constraints of finances and natural law.

One of the common dynamics in these warring couples is what I term the "need to be right." This need is often expressed by getting in the final word, or by the kind of verbal defensiveness that I have come to call "jousting," where nobody ever listens and no one ever really wins. The need to be right is ubiquitous, I think. I view it as a fuel that quite effectively feeds our denial. To me, the need to be right is one of the great enemies of recovery. It is a terribly dysfunctional attitude. Many who come at recovery with the need to be right will turn and walk away from this program as disappointed as the rich young ruler in the New Testament who once heard Jesus weave a bizarre tale about a camel struggling to squeeze its hump through the eye of a needle.

What I believe we are after when we want grace but when we are still unwilling to give up our need to be right is what Christian martyr and noted twentieth-century theologian Dietrich Bonhoeffer called "cheap grace." The following are his words:

Cheap grace is the deadly enemy of our Church. We are fighting today for costly grace.

Cheap grace means grace sold on the market like cheapjacks' wares. The sacraments, the forgiveness of sin, and the consolation of religion are thrown away at cut prices. Grace is represented as the Church's inexhaustible treasury, from which she showers blessings with generous hands, without asking questions or fixing limits. ...grace without cost...

Cheap grace means grace as a doctrine, a principle, a system. It means forgiveness of sins proclaimed as a general truth, the love of God taught as the Christian "conception" of God. An intellectual assent to that idea is held to be of itself sufficient to secure remission of sins....

Costly grace is the treasure hidden in the field; for the sake of it a man will gladly go and sell all that he has....

Costly grace is the gospel which must be sought again and again, the gift which must be asked for, the door at which a man must knock.[7]

Step 5: I admit my wrongs.

I have decided that the cost of grace in my own life is, among other burdens, my need to be right. That is exactly what grace has cost me—the denial of my own sin. Grace cost God God's own son. Grace, however, if I really choose to experience it, costs me the refusal to accept responsibility, which, of course, quickly unravels all manner of self-righteousness.

I cannot possibly work Step 5 and remain grounded in denial. Denial can be terribly expensive because ultimately this ugly defense mechanism, which I have honed for a lifetime, is precisely what I must swap for grace if I ever hope to experience any kind of genuine, lasting inner peace.

The simple fact is that I don't want to give up my denial. No, there is a rebellious, arrogant, narcissistic child dwelling in me who would much rather be right than peaceful. But there is also, thank God, a soul within this man who seeks peace and who longs to drop denial in the dust like a threadbare wool blanket and approach the throne of grace armed with nothing more than the willingness to confess the *exact* nature of his wrongs.

All of us are spiritual beings struggling to have a human experience. The woman who gave me this wonderful insight at a recovery meeting was absolutely right, and I have pondered her words many times. When I first heard her describe herself as a spiritual being struggling for a human experience, my thoughts turned to Vernon, whom I once knew in the context of the soup kitchen I directed in Dallas. I met him soon after another fellow and I founded the soup kitchen. Vernon had just been released from prison, and he had returned to Dallas, where he was to secure work and a place to live.

Vernon did neither, and he turned the time God gave him to live this life into nothing more meaningful than a long string of wasted days punctuated by obscene behaviors and bawdy songs that he sang loudly in the cause of offending as many genteel folk as possible.

In the decade I knew Vernon, I witnessed the deterioration of a man from a physically strong "cotton chopper," as he called himself, to an emaciated, pathetic figure with one leg. In our later years together, he was confined to a wheelchair.

On one already-hot August morning, I received a call from the folks in the Lone Star Gas Company Building, our neighbors in downtown Dallas. The call was actually a complaint regarding Vernon's "insufferable racket," as they termed it.

I felt no small amount of resentment welling in my consciousness as I pushed away from my desk and walked briskly through the door, where I happened upon old Vernon, drunk, of course, and singing as loudly as his lungs would permit as he sat slouched in his disgusting, urine-stained wheelchair.

I tapped his shoulder lightly. He glanced up at me and with slurred speech said, "Howdy, Bob. C'mon and sing a song with me."

I declined his offer as I began to push his wheelchair toward what shade a stand of live oak trees might provide him on the east side of the church. And as I rolled his chair beneath words covered in gold leaf carved in the granite lintel of a Presbyterian church proclaiming to anyone who might notice that "God Is Love," I suddenly recognized the song that Vernon sang. It bothered me some that I had even paused long enough to pay attention to this man who had suddenly become my responsibility.

He was singing "Nearer my God to Thee . . . Nearer my God . . ." with slurred speech and with an all-out butchering of the lyrics. But there in the sunshine, beneath the words "God Is Love," he sang one of the great hymns of the Christian church. And in that moment, I recognized this man for the very first time. Oh, his name was still Vernon, of course, but I recognized him by his real name—"Love." Obviously he had failed to acknowledge his own identity, just as most of us fail to acknowledge ours. But that was, and remains, his name—Love. It is each of our names, as well.

The choice for healing is always entirely ours. We can come to discover who we really are, but to do that, we must first approach a throne called grace and confess the *exact* nature of our wrongs to God. On the surface, this appears to be a simple Step. But the fact is, confessing the exact nature of our wrongs requires that we first make a commitment to care for ourselves.

Long ago a trusted and wise priest who was my dear friend offered me some sage advice: "Go ahead and confess your sins to God, and then be as gentle with yourself as you would be with a frightened child who you knew had no real reason to be afraid."

His words seem the most appropriate way to conclude any discussion on confession. So to borrow liberally from my friend, I would admonish you to confess, and then confess some more. In other words, take time with your confession and whisper to the child hidden deep within you that with your confession, you commit to loving that child with gentleness, reassurance, and the truth of God's grace.

Step 5: I admit my wrongs.

References

[1] Paul Tillich, *The Eternal Now* (New York: Charles Scribner's Sons, 1963), pp. 50–51.

[2] Ibid. pp. 103–104.

[3] M. Scott Peck, *Further along the Road Less Traveled*, p. 26.

[4] Ibid.

[5] Robert Bly, James Hillman, and Michael Meade, eds., *The Rag and Bone Shop of the Heart: Poems for Men* (New York: Harper Perennial, 1992), p. 195.

[6] M. Scott Peck, *Further along the Road Less Traveled*, p. 145.

[7] Dietrich Bonhoeffer, *The Cost of Discipleship*, reprint (New York: Macmillan, 1972), pp. 45–47.

6

Therefore be imitators of God as beloved children. And walk in love, as Christ loved us and gave himself up for us, a fragrant offering and sacrifice to God.

Ephesians 5:1–2 RSV

Step 6. *I am entirely ready to have God remove all these defects of character.*

This is what I call the "gettin' ready" Step. When I was a kid, I would join my brothers and cousins in playing a game of hide and seek. When "it" had finished with the ten count, he or she would holler in a voice louder than the first school bell of the morning, "Here I come, ready or not!"

Let us be clear at the outset: this is not some "ready or not" Step. No, this is a "ready" Step, and before you and I can get ready, it is always wise to consider the cost. In other words, if I am to work this Step, I see it as absolutely essential that I first recognize the payoff involved in my holding on to this disease tighter than a pair of rusty pliers.

"There can be no payoff," you say. "What could possibly be the positive payoff for hanging on to my drinking, drugging, unhealthy sexual behaviors, worry, control, dependency, gripping fear, obsessive thinking, compulsive behaviors, and life without boundaries?" Well, you may not pose the question in just that way, but, believe me, I have heard the question posed so often that I have come to regard it as the single most common interrogative associated with the whole process of recovery.

The payoffs are subtle; in fact, I suspect that they are far more unconscious than they are ever conscious. Two of the most common are (1) familiarity and (2) safety. In time, these two payoffs get so tangled up with each other that it becomes difficult to distinguish between them.

One of the most insidious facets of addiction is that it becomes very familiar. It doesn't take much time for me to learn how to become dysfunctional. I discover quickly how to live with the pain I suffer. Of course, this pain is anything but comfortable, much less comforting, but still, it remains familiar. And familiarity is a powerful force that should never be underestimated.

A few years back I was driving south on Interstate Highway 37 on my way to Corpus Christi when I spied, growing along side the highway, a clump of prickly pear, which of course is a beautiful, thorny cactus that is as ubiquitous in the Southwest as rattlesnakes and mesquite trees. I stopped the car and walked to the fence row, where I stood for a moment and admired the beauty in this particular clump of cactus standing taller than the highest strand in the barbed wire fence. I estimated the height of that tangle of cactus at more than five feet. That, even by Texas standards, is one tall old bunch of cactus.

Imagine, if you will, attempting to make such a cactus clump your bed. Further, if you will indulge my fascination with the absurd, fantasize that you have learned to contort your body every evening so that you might sleep in that cactus clump with the minimum amount of discomfort. Your bed is, of course, still terribly inhospitable, but the fact is that you have learned to sleep in it. As months turn to years, sleeping in cactus becomes, at first, simply what you know, and, later, *all* that you know.

Freeze that image in you mind and you hold a primitive, mental snapshot of precisely how this disease works. All over this globe, people daily make their beds in a metaphorical cactus clump. For a lifetime it remains, of course, uncomfortable, but it is what they have come to know. Sadly, many of them were told as children that a cactus clump is all that they deserved. Even more sadly, they believed it to be true then, and they hang on to that unexamined lie today. In a word, they have become very *familiar* with the notion that that prickly cactus clump is to be their bed. It is all that they know today and, for many, it is all that they have ever known or will ever know.

Now imagine that I walk up to your cactus clump one fine spring morning with the sky full of puffy clouds and the birds singing of the coming

Step 6: I am ready for the defects to be gone.

warmth and I offer you an invitation. Perhaps I begin with, "Hey, you don't have to sleep in that tangle of prickly pear. God has prepared a beautiful bed for you at the top of the stairs of a stately old house on the far side of yonder woods. This comfortable, soft old bed is covered with sun-dried linen sheets, and there is a light in the window and a fresh cup of hot chamomile tea waiting for you on the bedstand."

Common sense whispers to us that anyone in his or her right mind would jump quicker than a kangaroo rat at such an opportunity. Such, however, is seldom the case. I can tell you from years of counseling experience with those mired in the disease that folks simply *don't* jump at such an invitation. The reason for that resistance is the powerful force we know as familiarity. Familiarity is in this context a synonym for safety.

When I was in the milking pen assisting my granddaddy in the art of relieving our dairy herd twice daily of their burden of milk, he would often share with me all manner of proverbs that proved, I suspect, to be character-shaping aphorisms. One of my favorites was this: "The greatest risk is not risking." In my adult life I have heard it said by clients and colleagues as well that "wholeness is downright terrifying." And why is that so? Because wholeness is a path on which, most likely, we have never trod before. It is the only safe path, but for those of us who have never traveled it, in the beginning, it invariably feels very treacherous and unsafe. For many, it may feel perverse, bizarre, and even immoral. But no matter how it feels to us, it is always the right path.

Therefore, before we can work Step 6, we must first be absolutely certain that we are ready to crawl out of the cactus clump and endure the fear that invariably attends the arduous journey toward wholeness. In other words, to be ready, as the wording of Step 6 intends, we must to be willing to give up the sick payoffs of familiarity and safety that have kept us clinging for years to the habit of dysfunction.

When people say to me, "I'm ready for Step 6," I caution them to be very, very careful. "Are you ready to give up the payoffs of familiarity and your attachment to some sense of pseudo-safety?" I ask them. When they nod in the affirmative, I have one last question to pose: "And are you ready now to endure the fear?" If they nod again, I generally believe that they are ready to lift themselves out of the cactus clump and swap their preoccupation with familiarly and pseudo-safety for a sojourn down that terrifying, but redemptive, path toward wholeness.

Since I first read it, I have liked very much the following poem, entitled "Intimates," by D. H. Lawrence. To me, it illustrates concisely, in its abrupt style, the truth that the responsibility for love or wholeness, or anything else in my life *always* lies with me, never with anyone else:

> Don't you care for my love? she said bitterly.
>
> I handed her the mirror, and said:
> Please address these questions to the proper person!
> Please make all requests to headquarters!
> In matters of emotional importance
> please approach the supreme authority direct!
> So I handed her the mirror.

Essentially, what Step 6 means to me when I choose to take it is that I am now declaring, privately to God and publicly to people I trust, that I am *entirely ready* to, in the imagery of D. H. Lawrence, pick up the mirror, take a hard look at myself, and begin a new, healthy life of autonomy as opposed to clinging for one day longer to a dependency upon chemicals, other people, or sick behaviors. I am ready, even if I don't yet know how, to stand on my own two feet and to allow my unhealthy dependency issues to be nothing more than memories and tough lessons.

Step 6 is not one more lesson in psychological adjustment. I have decided that I have no interest whatsoever in being better adjusted to this culture. No, my investment through recovery lies far more on the side of learning and, more importantly, in practicing what it means to love. Therefore, I am not so much interested in psychological adjustment as I am in moving one step at a time, and one day at a time, toward the ultimate goal of my own spiritual maturity.

Step 6, then, is *not* a call to further psychological adjustment. Robert Linder offers strong insight into the problems we have caused in the lives of people by insisting that they "adjust":

> *You must adjust . . . this is the motto inscribed on the walls of every nursery, and the process that breaks the spirit are initiated there . . . Slowly and subtly, the infant is shaped to the prevailing pattern, his needs for love and care turned against him as weapons to enforce submission. Uniqueness, individuality, difference—these are viewed with horror, even shame, at the very least they are treated like diseases, and a regiment of specialists are available today to "cure" the child who will not or cannot conform.*[1]

Step 6 is about being ready for the giant step toward autonomy. What does it mean to be an autonomous human being? Marsha Sinetar provides a helpful picture of autonomy in the following description:

> *Each [autonomous and authentic person] has at least a high*

Step 6: I am ready for the defects to be gone.

enough degree of self-esteem that he is willing to act on behalf of what is, for him, real and worthwhile. Each also has the self-trust and self-reliance to know what he is about as a person, to identify—perhaps even to speak up for and act out—what is valuable, what he aspires to, what is meaningful. There are persons who have the necessary energy, determination and resourcefulness to assertively opt for a life they find worth living.[2]

For me, Marsha Sinetar has defined accurately the meaning of recovery in the phrase, "opt for a life . . . worth living." Step 6 is in my mind just that—the conscious decision to give up my neurotic payoffs for a life worth living. Again, a life worth living has nothing to do with being adjusted; it has everything to do with an autonomous sense of self that has willingly and consciously surrendered the ego in a dependent relationship only with God. Dependency upon God is the only healthy dependency in this life. What some term "interdependency," or the sharing of emotional support, talent, time, and love in a noncontrolling, conscious arena, is the mark of healthy human commerce, but again, the only healthy dependency that we human beings can have is upon God. Such autonomy, interdependency, and the faith to depend only upon God require courage.

Sinetar buttresses this point: "It takes high self-esteem and self-trust to sacrifice collective opinion, security, customs, guarantees in favor of that which one prefers and thinks is best. To sacrifice safe and direct routes of accomplishment—maybe even accomplishment itself as it is usually defined—also requires inner strength and faith."[3]

If you decide to work Step 6, don't expect your friends, or even members of your family, for that matter, to understand, appreciate, or applaud your decision to make the declaration that you are ready to have your character defects excised. It is quite likely that those closest to you will not understand, or even support, your courageous effort to have God remove your character defects. In fact, if you can expect any external forces at all, they will most likely arrive in the form of inertia and resistance. Many people will attempt to "seduce" you back into the mire, where they have learned to grow comfortable, and "dance," if you will, in your disease. In a very real sense, they have grown quite comfortable witnessing you sleep every day in a clump of cactus. Some may even have shared that metaphorical bed with you.

So it would be naïve to expect family and friends, or even the church, to support your recovery. No, the fact is that recovery can be terribly threatening to many such systems. For those of us who are willing to take Step 6, we must also be willing to go it, for the most part, alone. But in whatever we do, we always go with God and keep in mind that, when others abandon us, we always have the members of our recovery group to support us.

A big part of what it means to take Step 6 is an overt, conscious willingness to change the paradigms in our life. I have heard the same yarn spun in the many denominational settings in which I have served as a consultant for the past two decades. Each time the tale is attributed to the denomination of whatever professional or layperson who at the moment is "ragging" his or her own system. It goes like this: "You know, the seven [actually eight] great last words of Methodism, Lutheranism, Presbyterianism, etc. are these: 'We've never done it that way before.'"

That particular story is so threadbare that it scarcely brings even a chuckle anymore, but I fear that there is more truth in the tale than there ever was any humor. We human beings, in the church and beyond the four walls of the church, simply don't like change. It scares us. I don't know any better way of stating my own discovered truth about this.

As I have mentioned in earlier chapters, I served for ten years in a wonderful old downtown Presbyterian church in Dallas, where I assisted in the founding of a ministry to the city's homeless and poor. I am grateful to report that the work continues today. I was fortunate to be at the right place at a time in my life when I was filled with energy and a passion for doing what I termed "justice."

I had cut my theological teeth on the Old Testament prophets, and my biblical hero was that cantankerous old prophet from Tekoa, Amos. Therefore, I was not only determined to make my mark in Dallas, which in retrospect is evidence of my own unexamined, unbridled narcissism, but I was also committed to making a significant difference in the lives of those who suffered daily from the indignities associated with poverty.

I now see that what I attempted was close to impossible in one sense in that, far beyond my awareness, I was pushing the church to change the very core paradigms that many in the church had come to identify as their God. In other words, I spent ten years demythologizing their sacred institutions.

The more I pushed, the harder those folks in very subtle ways pushed back. I enjoyed a meaningful and, by any cultural measure of the situation, successful ten years with those Christians, but one day I quit. I knew that I was exhausted—burned out.

I accept full responsibility for my burnout; it was my own disease that caused me to push myself to the threshold of exhaustion. However, some years later I was visiting at dinner one evening with a seminary president

Step 6: I am ready for the defects to be gone.

from a distant state, and he commented that it must not have been easy working with the homeless for a full ten years.

I surprised myself by an abrupt assertion of what today I still perceive to be the truth. I said, "You're right. It wasn't an easy ten years at all. My real difficulty, though, lay not with the homeless folks. By and large, they were easy to work with. No, my problem was always with the church members. They were the difficult ones."

I believe the reason I suffered so in that job, in addition, of course, to my own disease, is that, right or wrong, I felt called to change the very paradigms of that particular old church. Such a conviction or sense of call is a setup from the beginning. There is no doubt that my narcissism was all tangled up in my theology, but the bottom line is that I burned myself out attempting to serve as a leader to people who did not demonstrate by one sign or wave of the flag that they were interested in changing the cultural paradigms of what a church "should be."

Step 6 is about the willingness to have God change the very paradigms of our life. I offer the foregoing story as evidence for the truth that you would be as unwise as a pullet jumping into the middle of a cat fight to believe for even one minute that you will get a whole lot of support when it comes to the business of changing paradigms.

Marsha Sinetar views emotional flexibility, or what I term the willingness to change paradigms, as a hallmark of what it means to be an autonomous human being: "If we cannot make it without old habits, toxic relationships, our addictions—whatever they might be—we are not free to choose our good. And while we are in the early stages of choosing that good, there is much to tolerate which calls for adaptability."[4]

To go at something as risky as change, I need a guide. I cannot do this alone, and, of course, the guide I am given for this journey is none other than the creator of the universe and the unconditional lover of my soul. What more could I possibly need?

At this juncture people occasionally ask me: "Do I have to know my character defects in order to be ready to have God remove them?" My standards answer to this is "Yes and no." Someone who has accomplished effective 4th and 5th Steps will probably possess a pretty good hunch as to the nature of personal character defects. For this person, the answer is "Yes."

If, in the course of my own recovery, I have identified my narcissism, my passive-aggressive traits, my strong (and sick) allegiance to passivity, my proclivity for avoidance, and my penchant for an unhealthy dependency upon others, but I still don't know all there is to know, the answer for me is "No." If I should seek to know it all, I will likely slip back into my disease in that I will strive to recover "perfectly." No human activity, including recovery, can be accomplished perfectly.

If I have been sincere in Steps 4 and 5, I have, at some level, come to trust God to take care of that which I don't yet know about me. Most likely my defects will continue to reveal themselves.

There is no doubt in my mind that, even given the amount of therapy and recovery work I have accomplished in my own life, I have still successfully hidden some character defects from myself. Every time new symbols (or symptoms) slip into my life in the form of depression and anxiety, I treat these visitors as gifts of the spirit that have come to share with me even more information. Some, though certainly not all, of that information has to do with my character defects.

Instead of hating the pain and shaming myself for its presence in my life, as I did for decades, I have come to accept not only the pain but also the incontrovertible fact that the pain is, if I will so permit it to be, an avenue into my inner self. The pain is also a wonderful and wise professor in that it knows far, far more about my soul than I could ever make available to my conscious mind.

This is a long-winded way of saying, yes, I do need to know something about the exact nature of my character defects before I say to God, "I am now ready to have you remove them," but I do not have to know it all. The simple fact is that in this life I will never know it all. Perhaps this is what the Apostle Paul means to convey in the thirteenth chapter of 1 Corinthians, verse 12 when he writes, "In a mirror dimly, but then face to face."

This is a good a place to share the story of the Colorado cinnamon bear: For more than three decades she has remained for me a living definition of what true liberation looks like.

That old bear came to visit one summer long ago to offer, I suspect, to teach me what liberation looks like.

She appeared daily at our dining room window on most mornings during that summer for the purpose of scratching her rotund belly in slow, comical strokes. Once she was satisfied that her claws had sufficiently disturbed what had to be a whole herd of fleas, she would amble off into the mountains scavenging for berries and wild rhubarb.

I suspect that I could have grown to like her except for the fact that she considered it her duty to rob our garbage pit every evening. With the ease with which I flip an electric light switch, she would take one swipe at the 70-pound steel lid that covered the pit and send it sailing into the night shadows.

On more nights than I can remember, she would awaken me with the

Step 6: I am ready for the defects to be gone.

thud of solid steel striking granite. I would sit straight up in bed and send loud threats in her direction, all to no avail. She would then balance her 500-pound frame precariously on the edge of that garbage pit while she swung one huge paw in the direction of a day's worth of pancakes, vegetables, and pork chop bones.

That old cinnamon bear wasn't at all choosy. She simply flipped the steel lid whenever she fancied, helped herself to whatever she found in that pit, filled her sizeable belly with garbage, and then retired into the night until she appeared, once again, the next morning in our window so that she might rearrange her fleas.

On one particular morning, I walked to the garbage pit to replace the lid, which she had discarded beneath a small spruce tree. As I dragged the steel cover to its place, I heard a distinct grunt followed by a groan emanating from the direction of the garbage pit. I paused, listened, and heard the sound of something wild a second time.

I flicked on the outdoor lights of the bathhouse and returned to the edge of the pit. Much to my horror, I found myself staring into the pitiful eyes of the cinnamon bear. She was now lying on the messy floor of that garbage pit six feet below the surface of the earth.

I forsook my shower and immediately aroused my sleeping comrades; together we hit upon the idea of lowering a ladder into the pit. We did just that, and that terrified bear treated it with no more respect than a bucking bull gives a rodeo barrel. In a matter of seconds, the first four rungs on that ladder were nothing but splinters.

Next we thought of lassoing her with a cow rope and tying the end to a horse and then pulling her out of the pit with sheer force. The only problem was, of course, that we could find no one to volunteer either to ride the horse or to cut the rope once that bear was out of that pit.

In that it was my day off, I declined any further interest in the bear's dilemma and drove off to Estes Park to do my duty with a week's load of dirty laundry. By the time I returned to the ranch, one intelligent, not to mention assertive, young colleague had called the National Park rangers. Once those fellows were finished with their guffaws, they encouraged my friend to cut two soft aspen logs and drop them into the pit in the shape of an X. It worked, and by nightfall, the bear had climbed those crossed logs and liberated herself from the garbage pit.

Our liberation occurs in much the same way. We really can do no more than approximate what we need when we are languishing in the garbage pit of our disease, but, like the old cinnamon bear, we can, if we so choose, go to the cross and listen carefully to the only one who can get us out.

Love liberates us, but unless there is discipline there is no love. All too often we are taught in this culture that love is something other than discipline. It is not! Scott Peck offers what I believe to be the best "secular" definition of any I have ever encountered: "[Love is] the will to extend one's self for the purpose of nurturing one's own or another's spiritual growth."[5]

If the cinnamon bear had not been disciplined in the sense of cooperating with the cross, she would have died a miserable death in that stinking pit. If we are to love ourselves, or others, we must first stretch ourselves, and, of course, such stretching invariably involves discipline. In my mind, love is a strenuous, disciplined effort or it is not love.

The Apostle Paul's immortal definition of love is as follows (1 Cor. 13:4–7): "Love is patient and kind; love is not jealous or boastful; it is not arrogant or rude. Love does not insist on its own way; it is not irritable or resentful; it does not rejoice at what is wrong, but rejoices in what is right. Love bears all things, believes all things, hopes all things, endures all things." I invite you to ponder this passage for a moment, and my guess is that in this moment of careful attention to the Apostle's words, you will come to recognize that what Paul is asserting here is the very point that I offered in the previous paragraph: love is a strenuous, disciplined effort, or it is not love. Love is the stretching of oneself, and I cannot possibly begin to extend myself in the cause of love without first having made the courageous decision to stretch myself beyond my old paradigms. Such stretching requires courage, discipline, and, most of all, patience.

When you think about it, the whole notion of patience—Paul's first descriptor of love—is also a discipline. None of us are born patient. Quite the contrary. We come into the world squalling impatiently in the cause of getting our needs met. Patience is a skill that is learned. It is a discipline. We must learn how to discipline ourselves if we ever hope to be patient.

Kindness is also a discipline. We learn to be kind because when we are children there are (we hope) big people in our lives who model regularly what it means to be kind. But we are not born kind. No, we come into this world armed with a strong predilection toward narcissism because our very survival depends upon our being very self-centered. Narcissism is something we grow out of and replace with genuine kindness, among other virtues; therefore, kindness is also learned. It, too, is a discipline.

Every descriptor the Apostle employs is, in fact, a discipline; hence, love as a whole is also a discipline, or a stretch. The culture that reared me lied to me, however, and taught me—in fact, convinced me—that love

Step 6: I am ready for the defects to be gone.

was nothing more than a feeling. Love is not merely some cozy feeling. Love has never been a feeling. We experience many feelings when we choose to love, but as Scott Peck writes, love is not a feeling.[6]

Love is a decision to live with a new sense of commitment to a disciplined life. If I choose to love, then I also necessarily choose to be disciplined. The inverse, however, is not necessarily true. I am acquainted with many folks who know what it means to be disciplined, but they have no real experience with love.

It is the love of God that liberates me from the garbage pit of my disease. But for that love to prove fully efficacious in the context of my healing, it is wholly incumbent upon me to cooperate fully with God by standing knee-deep in a small mountain of rotting muck and declaring to God that I am *entirely* ready to have God get me out of there. Such an assertion is, I believe, the very essence of Step 6. It is tantamount, I believe, to proclaiming, I am now *entirely* ready to have you remove these character defects. I am now *entirely* ready to cooperate with you. I am *entirely* ready to change the dysfunctional paradigms that rule my life. I am *entirely* ready for you to love me. And I am *entirely* ready to enter into the difficult discipline that is this thing I have learned to call love. For me, this is a snapshot of what it means to work Step 6.

Like all 12 of the Steps, this one also requires a wagonload of old-fashioned moral courage. Writer and prophet Will D. Campbell weaves tales with more passion than any living writer I read today. He was the single Anglo involved in the founding of Martin Luther King's Southern Christian Leadership Conference more than three decades ago. In his role as preacher and civil rights activist, he witnessed many acts of impressive moral courage, which he recorded with a rare and gripping flair.

The following story of a man's courageous decision to live the discipline love requires is contained in Campbell's *Forty Acres and a Goat*. The book treats the courageous, and all too often, bloody battle black people waged in this country to gain their civil and, according to our Constitution, God-given rights:

One school was destroyed by a dynamite blast in a nocturnal act of defiance. Nine days after the first black child had crossed its portal.

One of the children was the daughter of Pastor Kelly Miller Smith. Late one night I sat with him in his study, peeking often through the window in a vigil against threats to the building. After a long period of comfortable silence, I asked, "Kelly, what if something happens to little Joy?" He moved the candle, the only light we had risked, closer to him and opened his study Bible and began to read about Abraham being told by the Lord to take his only little boy up on a mountain, tie him on a pile of wood, cut his throat, and burn him. He read a sentence and then talked about it.

"Take now thy son, thine only son Isaac, whom thou lovest, and get thee into the Land of Moriah, and offer him there for a burnt offering upon the mountains of which I tell thee of."

"You see, my brother, we don't even get to choose the mountain," he said, "God chooses the mountain. All we're asked to do is obey."

"And Abraham built an altar there, and laid the wood in order and bound Isaac his son, and laid him on the altar upon the wood. And Abraham stretched forth his hand, and took the knife to slay his son. . . ."

I thought he was going to cry as he half closed the book. Instead he began to laugh.

"Will, we are talking about some hard sayings. We're talking about faithfulness to Almighty God. The God of Abraham, Isaac, and Jacob. The God of my black mama and daddy in Mississippi and your white mama and daddy in Mississippi. If that God says we've got to do it, we've go to do it. . . ."

I sat silent, a little sorry I had asked the question but grateful for the preaching. He put the Bible down, cast a quick glance out the window, then looked straight at me and quoted the rest of the Scripture from memory.

"And Abraham lifted up his eyes, and looked and behold behind him a ram caught in a thicket by his horns."

He leaned back, shoved the candle between us and bent his head in prayer: "Lord, make the thicket tight the ram's horns long. . . . Amen."[7]

Every time I read this story, I am reminded of Step 6, because it is in this Step that we are also talking about some mighty "hard sayings," to employ the words of Pastor Kelly Miller Smith. Anyone who tells you that it does not require courage to stand before God and declare, with a deep sense of reverential sincerity, the readiness to have one's character defects removed is mistaken and has, quite likely, never made anything close to such a courageous stand. Step 6 requires, I believe, the same fortitude that was required of Pastor Kelly Miller Smith when he decided to send his precious daughter into a public school filled with hate.

Any promise to God requires courage. Make no mistake about that. But even when I choose to be courageous, and when I choose the discipline of love over remaining asleep in a clump of South Texas prickly pear, the questions seem to remain and doubts seem to taunt me like

Step 6: I am ready for the defects to be gone.

circling buzzards.

In seminary I was delighted to discover the writings of Dietrich Bonhoeffer. Today, fifty years following his death at the hands of the Nazis, he is regarded as one of the most influential Christian thinkers of our time. If any man in this century dared to stretch himself in the cause of love, this man did. And if any man deserves a hearing, it is Dietrich Bonhoeffer, who refused to capitulate to Adolph Hitler, who refused to belong to any Lutheran denomination that would place the flag of the Third Reich in its sanctuary, and who courageously founded an underground seminary where he might continue to train candidates for a proclamation of the Gospel of Jesus Christ in a culture gone insane.

Even with a lifetime of demonstrated moral courage, Bonhoeffer doubted. Even in the wake of his adamant resolve to remain obedient to the God of Scripture as revealed in Jesus Christ, and to frame his obedience in the context of all that it could possibly mean for one to surrender completely to the will of the Almighty, Dietrich Bonhoeffer struggled with an enormous, almost unbearable, internal pain.

What remains so terribly impressive to me is that through it all, he was willing to write about his doubts and, even more, to share his most intimate journal entries with the world. The following poem is one such journal entry smuggled from his prison cell prior to his death:

> Who Am I
> Who am I? They often tell me
> I stepped from my cell's confinement
> calmly, cheerfully, firmly,
> like a Squire from his country house.
> Who am I? They often tell me
> I used to speak to my warders
> freely and friendly and clearly,
> as though they were mine to command.
>
> Who am I? They also tell me
> I bore the days of misfortune
> equably, smilingly, proudly,
> like one accustomed to win.
>
> Am I then really that which other men tell of?
> Or am I only what I myself know of myself?
> Restless and longing and sick, like a bird in a cage,

> struggling for breath, as though hands were compressing my throat,
> yearning for colours, for flowers, for the voices
> of birds,
> thirsting for words of kindness, for neighbourliness,
> tossing in expectation of great events,
> powerlessly trembling for friends at an infinite distance,
> weary and empty at praying, at thinking, at making,
> faint, and ready to say farewell to it all.
>
> Who am I? This or the Other?
> Am I one person to-day and to-morrow another?
> Am I both at once? A hypocrite before others,
> and before myself a contemptible woebegone weakling?
> Or is something within me like a beaten army
> fleeing in disorder from victory already achieved?
>
> Who am I? They mock me, these lonely questions of mine.
> Whoever I am, Thou knowest, O God, I am thine![8]

What a gift this man has given our undisciplined world. Nowhere in all the books and articles I have consumed both in the context of my own study for the ministry and on the path to my personal healing have I discovered a more rigorously honest statement of precisely what Step 6 is about. To me, Step 6 is essentially what Bonhoeffer has done so eloquently in this poem: stand before God with honest questions and then surrender with these or with similar words: "Whoever I am, Thou knowest, O God, I am thine." Such a confession, and such an acknowledgment, is, in my view, the fullest possible expression of what it means to be a spiritually mature human being. Another helpful way of looking at Step 6 is to view it as a deliberate, courageous Step out of a lifelong habit of some kind of entrenched infantilism toward what it means to be whole.

The Apostle Paul equated immaturity with ordinariness. There can be some strong argument, I suppose, made for such a claim in that immaturity is so ubiquitous as to be the norm rather than the exception. Therefore I wholeheartedly agree that what it means to be "ordinary" in today's culture may very well be synonymous with spiritual immaturity.

The following is Paul's view on the matter of maturity (1 Cor. 3:1–4): "But I, brethren, could not address you as spiritual men, but as men of the flesh, as babes in Christ. I fed you with milk, not solid food; for you

Step 6: I am ready for the defects to be gone.

were not ready for it; and even yet you are not ready, for you are still of the flesh. For while there is jealousy and strife among you, are you not of the flesh, and behaving like ordinary men."

Marsha Sinetar provides a compelling twentieth-century view of the immature personality. Her insight is no different from the description the Apostle provided twenty centuries ago:

The immature, underdeveloped personality is impulsive, opportunistic, and self-involved. In the mature human, greed and self obsession have given way to generosity, selflessness and a disciplined will that can give to others. When we speak of "arrested development" in people, we mean adults whose grown-up bodies actually are housing children. These are persons who, despite advanced chronological age, see narrowly, perhaps in an infantile way, are emotionally blocked or rebellious, and are fixated—stuck—when they encounter obstacles or problems in life. Some experience that should have been dealt with and assimilated was repressed into the unconscious realm of the personality, leaving the individual neurotic because he is still responding to life, and trying to solve his daily problems, out of the framework of infantile perceptions.

For the immature personality, fear is often a prime motivator for right action. Rules, laws, restrictions, and the threat of punishment for forbidden actions are all ways to insure that the individual controls himself.[9]

The question now begging for an answer is, of course, what does the mature person look like? I offered the best example of the mature personality in chapter 2, when I invited you to go back and study the personality of Jesus as you find him described in the four Gospels. In his thinking, his teaching, and most of all in his behavior, you will, without a doubt, discover what maturity looks like. The foremost feature in his personality is, of course, his adamant willingness to love. It is this very willingness to stretch ourselves to love that almost mysteriously shepherds us out of our immaturity, through the fog of our existential fear, toward what it means to be whole. Love is invariably a stretch. Love is also discipline, and love always begins with a commitment.

Goethe writes:

Until one is committed, there is a hesitancy, the chance to draw back, always ineffectiveness. Concerning all acts of initiative (and creation) there is one elementary truth, the ignorance of which kills countless ideas and splendid plans: that moment one definitely commits oneself, Providence moves, too.

All sorts of things occur to help one that would never otherwise have occurred. A whole stream of events issues from decision, raising in one's favor all manner of unforeseen incidents and meetings and material assistance, which no man could have dreamed would ever come true.

> Whatever you can do,
> or dream you can, begin it.
> Boldness has genius,
> power and magic in it.

An old man in East Texas once said to me when I was a child, "You know, you can't hardly steer no truck 'less first it's movin'." In his own way, I do believe that this octogenarian, who had probably never finished the third grade, and Goethe were saying essentially the same thing. There is, indeed, genius in boldness.

Step 6 is the Step of boldness, and of genius, and of power, and of mystery. Take it easy, but if you're entirely ready, take it.

References

[1] Marsha Sinetar, *Ordinary People As Monks and Mystics: Lifestyles for Self-Discovery* (New York: Paulist Press, 1986), p. 135.

[2] Ibid, p. 137.

[3] Ibid.

[4] Ibid., p. 138.

[5] M. Scott Peck, *The Road Less Traveled* (New York: Simon and Schuster, 1978), p. 81.

[6] Ibid., p. 116.

[7] Will D. Campbell, *Forty Acres and a Goat: A Memoir* (Atlanta: Peach Tree Press, 1986), pp. 51–52.

[8] Dietrich Bonhoeffer, p. 15 (Dietrich Bonhoeffer's poem "Who Am I" is used with permission.

[9] Marsha Sinetar, pp. 54–55.

7

Blessed are the meek, for they shall inherit the earth.

Matthew 5:5 RSV

Step 7: *I humbly ask God to remove my shortcomings.*

Five years following my ordination as a Presbyterian minister, I was invited to attend a Synod meeting, a gathering of the ministers and appointed laypersons from a four-state area. I traveled to this meeting with a saint of a man who possesses in his little finger far more patience about these kinds of matters than I will ever know.

This was to be a three-day meeting dedicated to committee reports, the approval or disapproval of all manner of esoteric ecclesiastical matters, and just plain sitting in an opulent Houston sanctuary. I call that sanctuary's style "rambling ranch house American colonial." Suffice it to say that the entire church was as posh as it was expansive. The building seemed to serve as sturdy testimony to its members' convictions regarding ensconcing themselves unashamedly in luxury.

For one full, tedious day I sat in that sanctuary and voted. Sometimes I would vote "Aye" and at other moments, just to break the monotony, I voted with a resounding "No!" Until that Synod meeting, I had regarded myself to be a somewhat intelligent man, but the fact is that through the whole of that day I never did comprehend either the import or the ramifications of those serial votes. No, all that I came to realize in that sanctuary was that I was bored.

The second day, I found it difficult—in truth, close to impossible—to shuffle once more to my place in that sanctuary. I lingered outside the mammoth church and savored a morning breeze that, I suspect, was about as fresh as Houston ever experiences. And for no other reason than that most any option appeared superior to further "participation" in the Synod meeting, I caught a city bus.

As I stepped aboard, I inquired of the driver as to the destination of the bus. He grinned as though he recognized my question to be as dumb as he must have figured I was naïve, and he mumbled from a behind a toothpick dancing about on his bottom lip, "To the end of the line."

"Does it come back here?" I asked.

"Sure does. Just as soon as it gets to the end of the line, I grab me one hot cup of coffee, and I drive this stinkin' bus right back to this curb as regular as some grandfather clock."

"Perfect," I thought. "Perfect! I am going to explore Houston, and no one in that sanctuary will even notice that I am 'absent without leave.'"

The ride proved interesting, in fact, fascinating. We passed stately homes and small glass and steel office buildings looming seemingly out of nowhere in a neighborhood where the landscape appeared far more suited, in my estimation, to the establishment of a park or the erection of even more housing for this obviously prosperous population.

I was impressed with the number of churches. None appeared as resplendent as the one I had abandoned, but there were plenty of them along that drive and most of them appeared, at least from the outside, to be doing what my granddaddy described as a "land office business."

The scenery changed abruptly. Where there had been signs of prosperity, the signals became very different. Through the bus window and over the dull roar of air conditioning, I could hear an occasional rumble from some juke box intent upon filling the late morning air with what sounded to me like vintage James Brown. Taverns, strip joints, pawnshops, and so-called convenience stores covered in steel bars suddenly became the norm. The bus stopped more frequently now, and the seats filled up around me with people of color.

Soon there was no place remaining to sit save the vacant plastic chair next to me. The bus jerked to a stop and an old man carrying a cardboard box obviously loaded with, what for him, was a week's worth of groceries slowly boarded the bus. He shuffled down the aisle as the bus rolled forward even before the door had completed its raspy wheeze.

I stood and motioned to this old African-American man who appeared to have celebrated at least his eightieth birthday. The old gentleman offered an obsequious smile that spoke more of a deep-seated fear, I sus-

Step 7: I humbly ask God's help.

pect, than of any real sense of relief.

He shuffled toward me on spindly legs and slipped slowly into the seat closest to the window as I held his box containing oatmeal, bananas, and staples.

We rode together sharing the same plastic, patched bus seat in near silence. Because I am often as driven by curiosity as I am fear, I had to know. Finally I posed this question: "Sir," I began, "for the past couple of days I've been meeting with some Presbyterians over in a big old church downtown. I wonder if, in your opinion, our meeting is making any difference to the folks who live in this neighborhood?"

The old gentleman stared straight ahead, obviously troubled by my question and, no doubt, wondering how he might answer in a manner that would subject him to the least amount of abuse.

As I slipped toward feeling guilty for having imposed upon his easy peace with the afternoon, he surprised me with an answer. In a soft voice he said, "I couldn't say, Suh, I couldn't say."

Hours later the bus driver kept his promise and dropped me off at the curb contiguous to the rambling ranch style colonial Presbyterian church. A fellow I shared a year or so with in seminary was standing alone on the front steps pulling frantic drags from what appeared to be a recalcitrant cigarette. As I approached the church's front steps he yelled to me, "Hey, Lively, you better get in here this minute. We're about to take one very important vote."

I answered, "Roger, I just discovered on that bus that what we're about here really makes no difference!"

He flipped his cigarette to the concrete, ground the butt beneath the sole of his tasseled loafer, and glanced in my direction long enough to bark, "You haven't changed a bit, Lively. You're still one crazy fool."

More than once I have heard such a description hurled at me, and I have come to believe that my critics are right. I am, in fact, crazy—insane is actually a more accurate descriptor of my true condition. But on that day years ago, I was not too far gone to realize that, for a few brief minutes on that bus, I had been in the presence of humility. What I discovered on the seat of that city bus was precisely that quality that was missing from our ecclesiastic meeting, and that all too often is absent in the church, as well: humility.

Step 7 is the Step of humility. It is the Step where I, with *disciplined* intention, begin the daily practice of humility. Like every one of these Steps, the practice of humility takes time. We can no more hurry it than we can hurry the composition of an artistic masterpiece. The practice of humility also takes effort, and it invariably requires the first descriptor the apostle Paul employed in offering to the ages the most insightful definition of love ever written. And what was that descriptor? Patience.[1]

Patience is the handmaiden of humility. One is virtually impossible without the other. I cannot be patient without first deciding to be humble, which, of course, requires putting my own ego on the back burner as I stretch myself for the highest good and the greatest growth of myself and/or of another person. And I cannot possibly be humble without being patient with the fact that it is terribly difficult, as well as emotionally taxing, for me to trust enough to sweep my own ego off center stage.

The reason this sweeping of the stage is so terribly difficult for me (us) is that I have been trained from the moment of my birth, perhaps even as far back as my conception, to survive in a culture in which the ego is lord. I reside in the culture of the ego.

Vince Lombardi, the immortal coach of the Green Bay Packers, is credited with saying, "Winning isn't everything. It is the only thing." Such thinking, while rather exciting and glamorous at first glance, is thinking born of the ego. It is but one of the tenets of this ego-centered culture that are working insidiously to shape our attitudes about life and even our faith.

If it is true that winning is the only thing, what church would aspire to swap opulence for sacrifice, and conspicuous consumption for genuine humility? Even the church has for twenty centuries been affected by the cultural forces grounded in the ego or in the strong emphasis on winning. However the word "triumph" is defined in each particular context, from the glitz of professional football to the orchestrated passion of professional religion, today's pastors are, in the main, every bit as dedicated to winning as any coach I ever met.

Will Campbell's tale of the racist and the plowman is a classic, and humorous, illustration of a head-on collision of two men both of whom were dedicated to one thing—winning. The following is a paraphrase:

> *An old black man is plowing behind a mule in the Mississippi Delta one fine spring morning when a young white man, who is obviously more full of himself than he is possessed of any kind of sense, brakes his Cadillac convertible to an uneasy idle on the dirt road adjacent to the plowman's field. The man in the Cadillac yells, "Hey, boy, how far to Jackson?"*
>
> *The black man continues to trudge behind the mule and offers no acknowledgment whatsoever of the man's question. A second time the young man in the Cadillac barks his question, this time with even more of an edge in his impatience, "I said, hey boy, how far to Jackson?"*

Step 7: I humbly ask God's help.

The black man utters not a word and only continues his plowing, paying no attention whatsoever to the man in the Cadillac. The white man lifts a twenty-two caliber rifle from the automobile's backseat, aims carefully, and shoots one of the guide ropes off of the black man's shoulder. Still the black man remains defiantly taciturn.

A second time the young white man fires, this time knocking the second guide rope from the old man's shoulders, and the black man trudges forward in the mud, never once looking up.

Now frustrated, the driver climbs out of his Cadillac, squeezes himself through the rusty strands of barbed wire fence, and marches to the place where the old black man has pulled his mule to a dead stop. The incredulous young man leans directly into the sweaty face of the plowman and with a voice raspy with rage he screams, "I said, boy, how far to Jackson?"

The old man slowly reaches into the bib of his overalls and removes a pistol. He raises it to the now-trembling young man's face and whispers, "You ever kissed a mule's ass?"

"No," replies the younger man with a new found compliance riding in his tone, "but I have always wanted to."[2]

To me, the story is about as humorous as it filled with pathos. It illustrates as well as any anecdote I know the nature of this ego-centered culture. Regardless of the progress we may have realized in areas such as civil rights, the culture in which we reside and attempt to grow spiritually remains, ego upon ego, and force upon force. Most often, the one with the most force, or the last draw, as in the case of Campbell's delightfully humorous tale, is the one who wins. And remember, in this particular culture, which is the locus of our own illness and where we are today seeking to discover healing and spiritual maturity, *winning is still everything.*

In the context of healing, an ego-driven effort avails us little. No, humility is the single efficacious approach to God. If we approach God through the ego, or through our need to control, we will come up empty-handed every time. Such an approach is tantamount to dropping a shiny new bucket in a dry well. The bucket may look good and the well may seem promising enough on the surface, but the effort will avail us nothing but dust and disappointment every time.

Thomas Merton writes,

The joy of the mystical love of God springs from a liberation from all self-hood by the annihilation of every trace of pride. Desire not to be exalted but only to be abased, not to be great but only little in your own eyes and in the eyes of the world: for the only way to enter into

> *that joy is to dwindle down to a vanishing point and to become absorbed in God through the center of your own nothingness. The only way to possess His greatness is to pass through the needle's eye of your own absolute insufficiency.*[3]

The cultural admonitions against such dwindling down to a vanishing point and becoming absorbed in God through the center of my own nothingness, to paraphrase Merton, are as powerful as they are pervasive. If you decide to work Step 7, that is, if you decide to stand alone before the throne of grace and *humbly* ask God to remove your shortcomings, you will definitely be planing against the grain of this ego-centered culture. Folks will not understand such a decision nor will they appreciate this bold step in the direction of genuine humility

As I mentioned in a previous chapter, I encourage you not to expect family, friends, members of your Sunday school class or, for that matter, even your own pastor to be supportive of this new call to humility. The cultural norms seek to ridicule humility as weak when, in fact, it is the surest sign of one's mental health and what it means to be spiritually mature.

As it turns out, what the culture defines as weak, namely, humility and a life surrendered to God, is the greatest strength we human beings can ever realize. Through the cultural lens we continue to equate strength with force and power with coercion, but God continues to work miracles in the lives of those who have traded force for the admission of their own helplessness and coercion for a new cooperation with grace.

Jesus understood that humility was the single path to God. Even more, he lived it. He was the most humble human being who ever lived, and, therefore, it is not all that surprising that he was the most surrendered man in history.

Two thousand years ago, a man named Saul believed that he was merely traveling down a Syrian highway to an out-of-the-way place called Damascus, when in fact, he was journeying from ruthlessness to sainthood, and from the role of persecutor to the humble office of apostle. In his letter to the Church at Galatia (Gal. 5:22), Paul lists what he, in his own spiritual journey, has come to discover as the "fruits" that can come only from a deep relationship with God: "Love, joy, peace, patience, kindness, goodness, faithfulness, gentleness, and self control." This same apostle, who was once a sociopath riding toward Damascus, has now changed his name to Paul, and his single conclusion regarding these so-called fruits of the spirit is that "against such, there is no law."

In my view, each of Paul's so-called fruits is a synonym for what it means to be humble. Humble people are very loving in that they stretch

Step 7: I humbly ask God's help.

themselves for the highest good of those they profess to love. Humble men and women are also joyful, patient, kind, good, faithful, and gentle and stand in no need of external societal controls.

As I mentioned above, Paul writes that there is no law against these characteristics, or "fruits," as he calls them. What does he mean? We can only speculate, but my suspicion is that the real meaning is to be found in the truth that any decision we make for humility is a response to God's claim upon our lives as opposed to a cognitive decision to comply with some statute. At the moment I choose to approach God through the daily disciplines required of humility, or through the behavioral expression of the fruits of the spirit, I no longer stand in need of the law. This is, of course, not any kind license for breaking the law, nor is it offered as a bizarre rationale against being "law-abiding." What I mean to convey here is that, if I make the decision to be truly humble, I am from that moment forward governed by a "calling" far higher than any law. And this calling will not likely place me in conflict with any reasonable or humane law that this society might establish.

Therefore, our choice for genuine humility is the choice for a life in which the law is no longer relevant to us. This is not a life of chaos, nor is it a life of "law and order"; rather, it becomes a whole new existence of "love and order" in which our order is directed and governed by something dwelling in us and at the same time far beyond us. I can call it by no better name than divine love.

Once again, I encourage you to be careful in seeking cultural support for any new decision for humility. Unless folks in your support system have hit some kind of bottom on their own, they will probably not even begin to understand, or remotely appreciate, what it is that you are experiencing as you deliberately and arduously plane against the grain of this culture.

You will, however, not be without guides. Christ is the best guide I know. Not only is he the sanest man who ever lived, he is, in my estimation, the very incarnation of what it means to be humble. Who else would have the courage to proclaim publicly from a mountain top blessings on those who are "poor in spirit"? Who else would have the gumption to stand before the world and offer for all time blessings for the "meek" and the "peacemakers of this world"?

Another guide, and a hero of mine, is Henry David Thoreau. Near the end of his stay at Walden Pond he wrote these words:

> *I learned this, at least, by my experiment that if one advances confidently in the direction of his dreams, and endeavors to live the life which he had imagined, he will meet with success unexpected in*

common hours. He will put some things behind, will pass an invisible boundary; new, universal and more liberal laws will begin to establish themselves around and within him; or the old laws will be expanded, and interpreted in his favor in a more liberal sense and he will live with license of a high order of beings . . . In proportion as he simplifies his life, the laws of the universe will appear less complex and solitude will not be solitude, nor poverty poverty, nor weakness weakness.[4]

An important, even vital, resource in our decision for humility is, of course, to be found in your recovery group. The most important mark for inviting someone to serve as our recovery sponsor is humility. If a person is genuinely humble, you can sense it. False humility requires some time to read, so as in every other part of this program, here, too, I invite you to take your time in the cause of recruiting a sponsor to guide you in the direction of genuine humility as you work these Steps. By all means, choose someone who has been to the pit and who remains humbled by the experience. Do not choose someone who obviously needs and therefore uses the recovery group as the stage for the expression of unconscious narcissism.

Wisdom always lies in humility, and it takes time as well as patience to figure out who is truly wise and humble or who may be simply introverted. I have always been severely introverted. I now regard my introversion as another gift of grace in that it provides me with the arena for regular contact with the deepest part of my soul.

This is not to suggest that extroverts do not share such contact and its attendant insight. I simply do not know because I have never been an extrovert, but I do recall many times when people have confused my introversion with wisdom. I was not wise; I was simply quiet because I really didn't know what to say in a particular circumstance. Wisdom is not introversion. Introversion is just introversion. For me, it is simply a gift of grace. I fully suspect that many others have discovered the gift in it as well, just as extroverts have discovered their extroversion to be an equal, but very different, gift of grace.

The truth is that wisdom lies not in extroversion or introversion, but, rather, in humility. So when searching for a real, live flesh-and-blood guide, search for someone who (1) has obviously been to the pit and returned safely, and who (2) lives life simply.

Over the years I have sought and consistently found great comfort in the words of Brother Lawrence, who was a pot washer in a monastery in seventeenth-century France. His words are recorded in a small book he penned that is still in print under the title *Practicing the Presence of God*.

Step 7: I humbly ask God's help.

Brother Lawrence regards humility as fundamental to the spiritual life: "The most holy, the most general and the most necessary practice in the spiritual life is the practice of the presence of God, whereby the soul finds her joy and contentment in His companionship, talking humbly and lovingly to Him always and at all times, without rule or system, but particularly in moments of temptation, of trouble, of spiritual dryness, of revulsion, and especially when we fall into unfaithfulness and sin."[5]

It is so very simple, but through our attachment to the ego, and through reinforcement by a culture that lives and dies with the winning-is-everything attitude, we complicate it. Such complications preclude simplicity.

So if you really want to choose an efficacious guide, look for someone who lives life nearly as simply as did Brother Lawrence. This plain man never sought any kind of fame, but during his lifetime, he became known as the most "peaceful" man in the whole of France. How he held onto his dedication to a simple faith and to the simple life in the midst of a world clamoring to know him is testimony, I believe, to his wisdom. So when looking for a spiritual guide in this process of recovery, look for another Brother Lawrence. There are men and women out there who are seeking God very imperfectly. Any one of them might work quite well as a sponsor as long as you perceive them to be humble.

A few years back a buddy of mine, whom I will call Dan and who was also a former student of mine, called me from a midsized industrial city in the Northeast where he had made his home. Following his ordination, this gifted young man had become the pastor of a dying inner-city church and had worked with no small amount of commitment and diligence to help the discouraged folks of his congregation find some reason to "be the church" in a neighborhood more marked by decay and degradation than by any signs of hope.

In the course of his first several years of work, he, along with several other pastors in the community, founded a soup kitchen. The success of the soup kitchen was immediate, and my young, plucky, sometimes even cocky, friend Dan enjoyed some small measure of positive notoriety for his efforts.

He had called me many times over the years, but this particular call was different. His voice was weak and, from his tone, I deduced that the man had either been ambushed by the negative forces I knew to exist in his congregation or he had been whipped by life in general, or both. Before I could launch into the usual amenities, Dan tossed at me a question for which he knew I could not possibly possess the answer: "Reckon who my AA sponsor is?"

I answered, of course, "Dan, you know full well that I have no more idea than a possum who your AA sponsor is."

I could hear him chuckling on the far end of the line as he offered me a twist of irony that to him proved so hilarious as to cause him to cackle. He continued: "My AA sponsor is a man I once lifted out of the gutter and fed meals to three times a day in the church's soup kitchen."

I decided that a protracted silence was the best course to pursue with young Dan. He continued, "When I finally got fired at the church for drinking, no human being in either the congregation or in the denominational office called to check on me. Not one! Can you imagine that?"

I could, of course, but I remained convinced that silence was still the best course.

"So, I'm suddenly jobless, penniless, stuck up here in some 'foreign' state that I wish the hell my ancestors had of whipped back at Gettysburg, and I don't know what else to do but to go to an AA meeting. So, I stumbled in drunk. Can you imagine going to an AA meeting drunk?"

"You're not the first, I suspect," I said, finally deciding to break my contract for silence.

"I kept going back. Finally I quit going back drunk, and one day, what those folks were up to in that 'church' began to make sense to me. I call AA my church, Bob," he explained.

I chose silence a second time.

"Finally, one day I decided to ask a young man, a black guy, to be my sponsor. When I first laid eyes on him, he did not look familiar. But the more I began to study this simple man in the meetings, the more I recognized that he looked familiar to me.

One evening, I mustered the courage to walk up to him and introduce myself. He grinned and said, 'I know you, man. You used to serve me meals in the soup kitchen. In fact, you were the one who picked me up out of the gutter. I've known who you were since you stumbled into the very first meeting drunk.'"

I interrupted Dan's story by laughing into the telephone.

He, of course, inquired, "What's so damn funny?"

"God's sense of humor," I answered.

Dan now barked at me: "But wait. This is the best part. This guy, who is my sponsor, says to me on that first day of our initial conversation in the AA meeting, 'Hey, man, you don't know God; you think you do. But the truth is that you don't!'"

"At first, I was furious with the bastard. Who is he to tell me that I don't know God. I've been to a seminary. Hell, I even learned to read the

Step 7: I humbly ask God's help.

Bible in the original languages long enough to pass the finals in Hebrew and Greek. I even have, or had, a Master's of Divinity degree hanging on my wall along with my certificate of ordination."

"I'll bet that impressed him," I cracked.

Dan laughed, "Yeah, about as much as it impresses me, anymore. What I finally figured out, and it took me months to do so, is that I didn't know anything about God. I wasn't humble. I was an arrogant, self-serving bastard. God to me was nothing more than my own sick agenda, my own chasing after recognition. That was my god. God to me was nothing more than my own career. God to me was how many people I could impress. God to me was nothing more than how much praise I could kick up for myself. God to me was nothing more than my own ego. I never realized that until I got drunk, stumbled, and eventually tumbled into the same gutter from which I once extricated the very man who has now graciously agreed to be my sponsor."

I said to my friend Dan, "God has been all of those sick things to me, and more. In telling me your story, you're telling me mine."

Dan remained unfazed by my close identification with his dilemma and he continued with a new urgency: "I have found God. But I didn't find God where I had always looked for him, but, rather, I discovered God in the darkest night I have ever been called upon to endure."

"I've lived one or two of those nights myself," I thought as Dan continued.

"And what I have discovered is that God calls us to true, not feigned, or artificial, but *true* humility before we can be of any real use to the Kingdom."

I include this anecdote in that it continues to serve me as a powerful teacher of the veracity contained in the words of Thomas Merton, I quoted at the outset of this chapter: "The only way to possess His greatness is to pass through the needle's eye of your own nothingness."

I know of no truer words. It is my impression, and nothing more substantive and empirical than that, that those of us who dot the landscape of this culture in the waning days of the twentieth century are so attached to the tenets of the cultural indoctrination in praise of the human ego that we must be "humbled" before we can ever hope to know what it means to be humble. Succinctly, we must hit some kind of *painful* crisis in our lives, where our own resources do, indeed, fail us, before we can come to comprehend that all along God has called us to a humble place where we have no choice but to ask God to remove our shortcomings. The simple fact is that I cannot remove my shortcomings. I do not possess such power, but God does and God will remove my shortcomings if

I will *humbly* ask.

This question emerges: What do we do, then, with the ego that we have worked on for a lifetime, hammering it, shaping it, polishing it, and bringing it to a fine, high-gloss finish? That question is crucial to any discussion of deciding for humility.

My conclusion is that we must give the ego away if we are to be healthy. That's right—we give it away. When we have developed some part of ourselves that is worthy of note, we give it away. When, for example, we gain the capacity to love with no strings attached, we give that love to others. When we learn to play the piano or the violin well enough to present recitals, we give our gift for music away to the world. When we learn to write, we write for the glory of God.

Once we develop an adult sense of self and when we come to know what it means to love with discipline, we are willing to give that sense of self to the highest cause of God's kingdom. This involves a process that is ongoing throughout the whole of one's life. Like love as defined by Paul, this process of developing and then giving away also never ends. I develop the ego, or my own sense of self, to one end, and for only one purpose—so that I may give it away.

Who gave us the gift anyway? God, of course. Therefore, my gifts are not my own. Whether they are developed or lie fallow somewhere, buried beneath layers of repression and denial, my gifts come only from God. Therefore, for me to claim credit, to take the glory, or to worship and praise my own ego is not only foolish, it is to overlook the obvious.

Everything belongs to God. In a very real sense, all of us are just what the man to whom I dedicated this book was: sharecroppers. Nothing belongs to us. We are mere stewards of the land, of our own lives, of our own gifts, and of all that which has been given to us. We commit a very serious error that can only bring upon us enormous grief when we perceive of ourselves as the authors or owners of anything.

What this book is about is my own attempt to honor God through the written word and through the process of giving my life away. I attended college once, I graduated from seminary twice, and I endured, as well as celebrated, two years in a counseling training program so that I might learn not only how to write, but what to write. This book is but one way I have learned to love through giving.

When I am healthy, I don't seek to give myself away because it brings me any personal gain. (Oh, to be sure, there is lurking in my soul an unrequited narcissist who loves the limelight attendant to publishing a book.) The only truly healthy reason for writing this book, or for listening to another human being's yearning for God, or for giving someone a sin-

Step 7: I humbly ask God's help.

cere hug, or for encouraging a brother or a sister who has fallen along the way, is that I have discovered that it is through giving my self away that I find my own life. I honestly can't explain it any better than that.

There is, of course, a paradox in all of this. The more I give away, the more I receive. I do not understand this, but then, if I did, it would cease to be what it is: a paradox. All I can suggest is that what I have discovered in my own life through the process of loving myself, or developing the ego for the sole purpose of giving it away, is precisely what Jesus Christ (Matt. 10:39) was referring to when he told us two thousand years ago that "he who finds his life will lose it, and he who loses his life for my sake will find it."

I suspect that the sole reason (except for the fact that I was already going bald) I never chose to become a hippie twenty-five years ago when I was in college, is that, deep down, I sensed that I really did not know what it meant to love. I was, if anything, put off by people my own age who staggered around Austin in those days, dragging on joints and offering the words "peace and love" to anyone who would stop long enough to hear such gibberish.

One of my all-time favorite tales illustrates this very truth vividly. It concerns Dr. Stuart D. Currie, the single Renaissance man I have ever encountered. He was the most brilliant scholar with whom I was ever privileged to study. In truth, his genius was exceeded only by his genuine humility. I have never known another human being, with the possible exception of this man's brother, who so closely walked the talk of God's love.

On a spring afternoon in the final semester of my senior year, Dr. Currie was ambling across the campus of the University of Texas, which is across the street from the seminary where he taught New Testament Greek Exegesis. Quite typically, he was engaged in reading his New Testament Greek text in route to a small grocery store where it was his daily custom to purchase a carton of buttermilk.

Suddenly, and much to his surprise, this eminent, but wholly unpretentious, scholar of the New Testament was delayed on the sidewalk by a young Christian zealot who was obviously out save this older man's soul.

He touched gently the crook of Dr. Currie's elbow and stepped back so that he might study this middle-aged gentleman now before him on the sidewalk dressed entirely in the type of khaki worn at the time by university maintenance crews. The zealot said, "Sir, I have two things to tell you. I love you and God loves you."

The professor paused, tilted his hat to the back of his head, and said, "Well, sir, half of that is good news."[6]

Humility is often difficult to understand in the context of self-love. Turning once again to the metaphor of the milking stool that I developed in an earlier chapter, the question before us is this: how do I love myself appropriately without permitting my preoccupation with myself (narcissism) to get in the way of what Step 7 requires, namely, a radical commitment to humility? Nowhere in all of my meandering in the literature of the field of pastoral counseling have I found a better definition of self-love than is located in William Miller's *Your Golden Shadow*. Miller maintains that appropriate self-love, among other decisions, is demonstrated by one's willingness to be assertive for oneself.[7] Being assertive for our own wants and needs is in no way antithetical to any commitment we might make to humility. In fact, the opposite is true. If I am assertive for myself, I will have no need to become aggressive, and it is this latter trait, not assertiveness, that proves to be the enemy of humility.

Aggression, the antithesis of assertiveness, is an intrusion, conscious or unconscious, upon someone else's ego and personal, spatial, or sexual boundaries. Aggression means to spill over my own boundaries like some lawless torrent and intrude upon the rights of other human beings. It is always a dysfunctional behavior in that it is invariably regressive, consistently manipulative, and often, if not always, grounded in beliefs that are far less than the truth.

Assertiveness is speaking the truth for myself from my own point of view with the hope that someone might hear me and respond. It is the expression of my humble needs within the context of my own boundaries. Simply because I choose to be assertive is no guarantee, however, that anyone will respond, but assertiveness is functional behavior in that it is predicated upon the truth as I perceive it.

Authentic humility is a decision and a commitment I make before God to live this life well. Authentic self-love is not gratification of the ego; rather, it is the development of a life worth giving away.

Ask yourself this question. Who is the most humble woman or man I know, or have ever known? Then, take the time, in the context of working Step 7, to list the qualities that point to humility in that individual. My strong suspicion is that, as you make your list, you will discover that each one of these people was deeply spiritual. Notice that I did not say they were religious; rather, they had surrendered their sense of self to God or, at the very least, to some sense of the transcendent.

In all of history I can think of no figure who was more humble than Abraham Lincoln. In his marvelous little book, *Abraham Lincoln: Theologian of Anguish*, Elton Trueblood writes of Lincoln:

Central to the new spiritual development was an enlargement of

Step 7: I humbly ask God's help.

the idea of vocation. Less and less did the President think that he was acting merely in his own will or depending upon his own meager resources. "Hate, fear, jealousy," as Sandburg put it, 'were rampant' in the summer [of 1862], but that was not by any means the total story, for Lincoln grew immeasurably as he came to think of himself as the 'instrument' of God's will. He needed an idea of this magnitude to keep him going in the face of unjust criticism as well as military defeat. The sense that there really is a Guiding Hand, which makes possible a genuine calling for both individuals and nations, gave a tremendous new sense of moral strength....

What was more important, Lincoln came to believe, was the effort to discern a pattern beneath the seeming irrationality of events. He had come to believe that God molds history and that He employs mortals to effect his purpose.[8]

Lincoln once wrote, "It is a momentous thing to be the instrument, under Providence, of the liberation of a race."

Whether we are president or an ordinary man or woman struggling to make it in this world, what was true for Lincoln—that he was an instrument of God—is also true for us. To recognize and to embrace that truth and then to live it out, *one day at a time,* is what it means to remain committed to Step 7.

But if I'm wandering around this planet wholly unsurrendered, struggling hard every new day to get *my* ego needs met on *my* own terms, I will never see myself as an instrument of much of anything other than my neurotic self-absorption.

We are all instruments of God. And as grandiose as such an assertion may sound on the surface, it is, in fact, a statement of genuine humility. When I finally decide to swap being the instrument of my own will for serving the higher calling of God, I swap narcissism for a genuine experience of surrendering to an intelligence who can do far more with this gift I call a life than I can even imagine.

Narcissism, then, is the grand impediment to Step 7, in particular, and to any kind of recovery, in general. In my view, the most dramatic characteristic of the narcissist is an adamant unwillingness to surrender anything. Scott Peck describes narcissism even more specifically: "Narcissism is the principal precursor of incivility. . . . One way to look at narcissism is to regard it as a type of thinking disorder."[9]

Permit me to illustrate what Scott Peck is describing here with an example from my own counseling practice. John Doe wandered into my office one summer afternoon, introduced himself, perched his body tensely on the edge of the sofa in my small office, and launched into his self-introductory remarks:

"Yeah, I hear you and I have a mutual friend . . ."

"Who is that?" I inquired.

"Why, it's old Joe Blow," he offered, still studying me carefully.

"I like Joe a good bit. In fact, I consider him a friend," I said.

John Doe replied to my recognition of the man. "Yeah, I like him enough when I need him for something."

Such, I submit is an unconscious disclosure of full-blown narcissism, the stumbling block to humility. At the core of narcissism is a deep-seated, unconscious pain that drives the narcissist toward an internally imposed sense of self-importance and grandiosity.

John Doe was, as I came to discover, "unsurrendered" and, as you can imagine, far less than humble. He was, indeed, quite narcissistic. By his report, his life was one miserable episode of "being misunderstood" after another. I was, I am certain, of little, if any, assistance to him, but we parted friends. I must report feeling terribly sad as he left my office perhaps more confused than when he came in.

Paul writes (2 Cor. 3:5): "Not that we are sufficient of ourselves to claim anything as coming from us, our sufficiency is from God, who has qualified us to be ministers of a new covenant, not in a written code but in the Spirit; for the written code kills, but the spirit gives life." Paul writes the truth. We are *not* sufficient in ourselves. We have never been sufficient in ourselves, and it is just as true that we will never be sufficient in ourselves, but don't tell a narcissist that. To the narcissist, the self, or the ego, is God, and to one who suffers from this disorder, humility is difficult at best and, in some cases, I suspect, even impossible. Humility is the single path to God because it requires that I surrender my false god of the vaunted ego to the true God of creation and redemption.

As I drive in my pickup through Central Texas, the capital of rugged individualism and the place in this culture where, I suspect, the Bible Belt buckles, I am often amused by the bumper stickers I see. One of the most revealing of the sickness that permeates our culture reads as follows: "It's hard to be humble when you're as GOOD as I am!" I know of no better declaration of the full meaning of narcissism than the words printed on that bumper sticker. Narcissism lulls us into believing the lie of our innate goodness and even of our own greatness. Narcissism confuses what it means to be created in the image of God with being God.

Of course, the truth is that I am not God. Being created in the image of God means that I am created with the potential to love. The bumper sticker is right about one thing, however. It is very difficult to be humble in this culture of the ego. The reason for that difficulty, however, lies not

Step 7: I humbly ask God's help.

in my capabilities or in my self-sufficiency, but in the simple fact that I, whether I am aware of it or not, am always afraid.

Step 7 is another in 12 simple Steps on the journey toward home. Coming home is the expressed hermeneutic of the amazing church where I now serve as a teacher and counselor, and it is also a solid theological perspective on what it means to be open to God's grace. For it is only when I begin chiseling away at my narcissism that I truly come home to my authentic self and also to God. The notion of coming home appeals to my soul as well as to my every conscious instinct. I connect to it, and its reassuring message resonates so deep within me that I cannot possibly connect descriptive language to the experience.

When I was fourteen, I wandered one late December afternoon into one of my granddaddy's pastures in search of whatever I might shoot at with the twenty gauge shotgun I had hoisted on my skinny shoulder. I felt like an adult, like a real man.

It was my first time to hunt by myself, and I savored being alone in the winter woods with nothing to keep me company but a dog named Pup and my burgeoning curiosity. To this day, I still do not know what happened, but somehow I managed to get lost. The next thing I knew, I was bewildered somewhere in a pine thicket belonging to either Mr. L. C. Henderson or to Ollie Hudson, both of whom were fence neighbors to my granddaddy. For the life of me, I could not figure out where I was. I knew that I was too old to cry, but I was also too frightened not to. As the afternoon sun began to sink over the tall pine trees toward the western horizon, I could sense a chill filling the coming darkness. I did not look favorably upon the idea of shivering away the night on a mattress of pine needles.

I knelt at the side of a creek and began to pray in earnest. I honestly didn't know what else to do. I had no sooner completed the first of what I was certain would be several "amens," when I opened my eyes to see my father and my grandfather walking toward me across a barren winter pasture. In my innocence I saw them as nothing less than the Trinity coming to carry me home.

Those two men hugged me and never once did they chide me or humiliate me for getting lost on my own land. Perhaps when they were but fourteen they had committed a similar error. I don't know about that, but what I do know for certain is that, because of love, those two men, along with a spirit, came to my lonely place in the mud for the sole purpose of guiding me safely home.

That is what Step 7 is all about. It is the willingness to drop to our knees in the mud in prayer and to say something like, "God, I don't know how to make it home. Please help me. I *humbly* ask you to remove my shortcomings. I cannot remove them, but I know for a solid gold fact that you can."

Three centuries ago, Brother Lawrence of the Resurrection wrote: "By this practice the soul comes to such knowledge of God that almost all her life is passed in making acts of love and worship, of contrition and trust, of thanks, of offering, of petition, and of all virtues; sometimes, indeed, she seems engaged in one unceasing, endless act, for the soul is keeping herself continually in divine presence."[10]

What more could we possibly ask for? What more could we possibly need?

This Step, like the others, is so very simple. I find, however, that chipping away at my own narcissism is mighty close to a full-time job that can be accomplished only one day at a time. I encourage you to go slowly with Step 7 and, above all, to be patient, very patient, with yourself. Coming home to God is never easy, especially if you've been away for a while. But you're on the right path. Its name is humility.

References

[1] 1 Cor. 13:4 RSV.

[2] Will D. Campbell, *Brother to a Dragonfly* (New York: Seabury Press, 1979), p. 136.

[3] Thomas Merton, *New Seeds of Contemplation*, p. 182.

[4] Henry David Thoreau, "From Walden . . . Conclusion," in *The Romantic Movement in American Writing*, Richard Harter Fogle, ed. (New York: Odyssey Press, 1966), p. 157.

[5] Brother Lawrence of the Resurrection, *The Practice of the Presence of God*, trans. Donald Attwater (Springfield, Ill.: Templegate, 1974), pp. 110–111.

[6] Thomas W. Currie, Jr., *The History of Austin Presbyterian Theological Seminary* (San Antonio: Trinity University Press, 1978), pp. 222–224.

[7] William A. Miller, *Your Golden Shadow . . . Discovering and Fulfilling Your Undeveloped Self* (San Francisco: Harper and Row, 1989), p. 110.

[8] Elton Trueblood, *Abraham Lincoln: Theologian of American Anguish* (New York: Harper and Row, 1973), p. 31–32.

[9] M. Scott Peck, *A World Waiting to Be Born*, p. 109.

[10] Brother Lawrence of the Resurrection, p. 126.

From now on, therefore, we regard no one from a human point of view; even though we once regarded Christ from a human point of view, we regard him thus no longer. Therefore, if any one is in Christ, he is a new creation; the old has passed away, behold, the new has come. All this is from God, who through Christ reconciled himself and gave us the ministry of reconciliation; that is, God was in Christ reconciling the world to himself, not counting their trespasses against them and entrusting to us the message of reconciliation.

2nd. Corinthians 5:16–19 RSV

Step 8:   I make a list of those persons I have harmed, and I prepare myself to make amends to them all.

This step occurs as a conscious response, as opposed to any kind of unconscious or emotional reaction, to our recognition of God as our authority. When I recognize, through the course of the previous 7 Steps, that it is God who calls me to a ministry of reconciliation, God who is the ultimate authority in my life, it is then that I realize that this Step must be accomplished. I have no other choice unless I continue denial and the "business-as-usual" approach that breeds the internal misery called despair. In fact, if I hold God to be the authority for my decisions, and if I still choose not to attempt reconciliation with those I have injured, plain old common sense demands that I excise the above-cited passage from the Scripture.

God has called me, and you, to a ministry of reconciliation. I cannot fail to act upon that mandate for reconciliation and still claim to be any kind of Bible-based follower of God. Also, without taking this Step (as well as the subsequent Step, which leads to the difficult measure of actually making amends), I will discover no lasting peace. The lens through which I view life will remain the same, and I will continue to regard men and women in the same old way I have always perceived other human beings. Because of this refusal to alter my perspective, I will invariably fail to recognize that those of us who claim the spiritual journey as our own, have had bestowed upon us a ministry of reconciliation. That ministry is *our* ministry; it is not an activity relegated to some paid religious professional. *The ministry of reconciliation is always ours!*

The fact is, when we accept the ministry of reconciliation, we may never again regard folks in the same old ego-centered manner. No, we will begin to regard them in a radically new way, and because of this dramatic, courageous shift in our perceptual paradigms of reality, we will, in time, experience more peace than we might ever have believed was possible for us.

The peace that arrives to comfort us, to guide us, to nurture us toward additional growth when we finally make the decision to trust God as our ultimate authority, and when we dare to shift our paradigms of reality from ego-centered to God-centered, or what I like to term "soul-centered," is truly amazing.

Thirty years ago, Truman Capote wrote a terrifying and chilling novel entitled *In Cold Blood*. This mesmerizing work was based on a true incident that involved the murder of four of the world's "salt of the earth" people, the Clutter family in Holcomb, Kansas, in November 1959. These gentle, responsible, church-going, ordinary people were shaken out of their sleep one dark night and murdered in cold blood for no apparent reason and with no obvious motive.

The murderers were two ex-convicts who successfully evaded the police until they were, months later, arrested in Las Vegas, Nevada. Several years passed and, after the trial, the convictions, and the standard appeals that invariably attend sentences of capital punishment, the two killers were sentenced to hang.

In Capote's book, one of the killers, a young, desperate man named Perry Smith, trembles at the foot of the gallows minutes before his execution:

Step 8: I prepare myself to make amends.

> *But after the warden asked if he had anything to say, his expression was sober. His sensitive eyes gazed gravely at the surrounding faces. . . . His assurance faltered; shyness blurred his voice, lowered it to a just audible level. "It would be meaningless to apologize for what I did. Even inappropriate. But I do apologize."*[1]

In a far less dramatic way, the message conveyed in that morbid scene is precisely what this Step is about. It is never meaningless to apologize. Step 8 requires that I list those I have injured, and I prepare myself, through the process of the prayerful surrender of my ego, to make amends to every name on the list of those whom I have injured.

Now is a propitious time for yet another word of caution. Remember that Jesus told his disciples that this is a world filled with wolves. Therefore, he admonished his own disciples to be "as wise as serpents and innocent as doves."[2] What this means to me is that there are some people I have injured who are not healthy enough themselves, in my judgment, for me to offer face-to-face, one-on-one amends. I may know from a previous experience that these people are so unhealthy, or even so ruthless, that it would neither be wise nor prudent for me to risk subjecting myself to any further abuse by presenting myself to them in person in the innocent context of making amends.

My advice to you is to follow the words of our Lord Jesus. If you know someone to be a "wolf," or if your intuition tells you that this person is unhealthy, then by all means be as wise as a serpent and as gentle as a dove. Write your apology to that person and mail it to God. Many of my clients have written an apology to some unrecovered, abusive person on a sheet of paper, stuffed it into an envelope, and mailed the thing to God by dropping it in a river, burning the envelope in a fireplace, or even mailing it through the U.S. Postal Service. (I've often wondered what the folks at the post office think when they receive an envelope addressed to God.)

You, of course, are the only one who can be the judge of who is a wolf. Please, however, be certain that you are not copping out by regarding the persons you fear as wolves. I believe that there are actually fewer wolves out there than there are people with whom we need to stand face to face, or to visit by telephone, or to communicate with via the U.S. Mail in the context of offering our apologies.

Another word of caution: do not expect the people to whom you make amends to be as healthy or as recovered as you are seeking to be. Most will not understand what you are up to simply because they are not, themselves, involved in any kind of disciplined recovery program. Some folks will, I suspect, even have their suspicions kicked up all the more in that you are, from their perspective, behaving in a bizarre way. They will not understand, so don't expect them to be empathic or receptive to your program of healing. A few will laugh at you and deride you, and some will even use the occasion to further "educate" you and inform you as to what an absolute fool you are. This last reaction, of course, borders on emotional abuse, so once again, I invite you to be judicious regarding to whom you decide to make amends.

Also, if in the context of an apology you sense that you are being abused, remove yourself gently from the situation, but by all means remove yourself immediately. Recovery is not intended to be a setup for further abuse. Offer a silent prayer for the abuser as you make your exit and tell yourself the truth—that your work with that individual is finished. God has forgiven you for the offense, and if the person you injured refuses to forgive you, there is nothing you can do. You and I are, remember, absolutely powerless over what any other human being does or doesn't do.

Some years ago in the context of my own healing, I wrote a letter to a former boss, a college president for whom I once worked. I informed him in this letter that my many conflicts with him were, in fact, little more than the projections of my own unconscious issues with authority figures. Further, I apologized for the hurt that I inflicted upon him and I reported that for the first few years following my departure from the college staff, I had characterized him in less than flattering portraits to mutual acquaintances and colleagues, the motive for my ugliness being that I had intentionally sought to injure him.

Some days later I received a letter back that did not truly surprise me. The man said he was, of course, aware of my less-than-kind remarks, and then the tone of the letter drifted off into some vague, harmless point that had nothing whatsoever to do with reconciliation. My point is that his response was not a letter of reconciliation in that he made no mention whatsoever of his part in the dysfunctional, less-than-peaceful relationship we shared for the nearly two years I worked under his supervision. He did not abuse me in his letter, but neither did he choose to be kind or conciliatory or to offer any real warmth. He is a gifted, even brilliant man, and what I said about him at one time, twenty years ago, is unconscionable. I made my amends to the gentleman, and he responded in the way that made sense to him, I suppose

For this program to work, that is all that must occur. I am not, nor are you, responsible in any way for the responses or reactions apologies generate in others. Therefore, when you are making your list and preparing your soul for making amends, discipline yourself not to expect a quid pro

Step 8: I prepare myself to make amends.

quo. The quid pro quo relationship is, of course, a this-for-that kind of interaction. If I give you this and in exchange you give me that, this is a quid pro quo transaction. Every time I walk into a store to purchase a soft drink, I give the person behind the counter about sixty-five cents. That person gives me the soft drink. That is an example of a simple quid pro quo transaction.

For us to expect some cozy quid pro quo relationship with people we have injured is highly unrealistic. These folks are far more likely to be resentful than they are to be in any way conciliatory. They are probably frightened to have us intrude upon their life again. After all, we did injure them, and once I have been hurt by someone, the last person I want to have any real commerce with is that individual who has done me some serious emotional damage.

So I don't blame the folks I have injured for being skittish, defensive, angry, projective, or whatever behavior they select to defend themselves. It makes perfectly good sense to me for them not to trust me. There is never any excuse for abuse, however, and while I should never consciously subject myself to such, I do need to be willing to take, and absorb, the heat that may accompany any significant effort at making amends. Therefore, in working Step 8, it is as natural as cold wind in winter to be nervous, edgy, and even more than a little frightened.

When I compile the list Step 8 requires, I inevitably kick up my own sore feelings and call forth, probably with a sense of righteous indignation, my own irrational "justifications" for my injurious behaviors. Those distasteful memories are merely a concomitant, or by-product, of this work. In my humble opinion, the reason we have Step 8 rather than just jumping out of Step 7 into the remainder of the program is because this Step provides us with an interim period during which we may make some kind of peace with uncomfortable memories.

Further, Step 8 guides us toward a radically new perspective or, as the apostle Paul put it, into a new way of "regarding" people that is free of the excess baggage of the need to be defensive, defended, or even "right." Such a shift in perspective takes time, and I would not want to launch into the actual making of amends without the preparation that this Step encourages.

Once we enter into Step 8, we come to recognize that none of the old ways of viewing reality seem to matter anymore. In recovery, I come to regard myself as a new creature. I no longer have to justify myself, as I have done for a lifetime, and it is no longer important that I be "right" or win an argument ever again. All that I must do today to continue on the journey toward the spiritual healing that brings the inner peace I earnestly seek is to prepare a list of those whom I have injured and be ready to make my amends. That is all that is required today.

If I get stuck in Step 8, it is most likely because my old view remains in control. It is this archaic perspective that is tied, inextricably, I fear, to some childhood introjection (learned internal message) that remains convinced that life *should* be fair.

If you believe that life should be fair, or even might, at times, be fair, you will encounter a major stumbling block in working Step 8. And if you hang onto the notion of the "shouldness" of fairness, you are also quite likely to get stuck in Step 8. The fact is, life is not fair. Let us get that straight from the git-go. *Life is simply not fair. It never has been, and I expect that it never will be.*

On a January 1 in the early 1980s, I opened the door of the church's soup kitchen early because the wind was whipping the streets and threatening frostbite to any who, by virtue of their tragic state of homelessness, might expose their flesh to the raw cold. I was particularly self-righteous that morning in that I was aware that I was bucking for special recognition in heaven, if not for all-out sainthood. The vast majority of the good citizens of Dallas were at home next to a warm hearth, and here I was alone, shivering with the homeless as I struggled against the elements to make these tragic figures safe and as comfortable as I could.

No volunteers had yet arrived to assist me. For reasons that remain unknown to me, except that schizophrenics are at times, and especially under stress, quite unpredictable in their behavior, an obese schizophrenic named Susan ambled to my station at the soup kitchen's front door and, without a word of warning, proceeded to dump the entire contents of a full ashtray upon my head.

I was furious—enraged is more like it. I hauled the enormous woman outside by the arm and left her to the cold until my friend, a true saint as well as a priest, arrived to calm me. Immediately, he welcomed her back into what warmth the soup kitchen might provide. I will never forget his words to me, "You've got to give up the notion that life is fair, Bob."

He was right, of course. I had in my anger abused the poor woman by pushing her away from me and into the icy wind and dangerously low temperatures. Thank God the priest came along. I am even more grateful that he confronted me in such a loving and powerful way. Life is not fair. I honestly didn't expect a thank you from Susan, but neither did I expect to be treated so harshly, in fact, abused by this disordered woman. But then she didn't ask for the disorder, and in that the schizophrenia plows so deeply into a person's ability to make

Step 8: I prepare myself to make amends.

good decisions, she certainly deserved grace rather than judgment, especially on such an inhospitable day.

Life is unfair. Sometimes we even get yesterday's cigarette butts dumped on our heads. There is no other reality that makes sense to me anymore. If I hang onto a passionate insistence upon making life fair, I remain, in reality, unconvinced that I cannot myself be God or the controlling authority over all human commerce. How absurd is this belief that underlies my behavior. I cannot possibly be God. Neither can I make life fair. All that I can do is love God, others, and myself and work to be spiritually mature and, therefore, peaceful.

What impedes us from taking Step 8? The same force that impedes us from taking any of the Steps or from spiritual growth in general: unconscious, unbridled fear. Marsha Sinetar paints a vivid and, for me, quite uncomfortable portrait of the fearful personality: "A fearful individual is a person held in check, stunted, even crippled—although his body may be perfectly formed. The longer the fear persists, the more he is stuck and frozen, passively unable to express what he needs or knows he wants. This type of fear can mask itself as anxiety, or as a disorderly, confused mind, incapable of thinking things through and incapable of identifying life-important answers."[3]

Traditional psychotherapy, or counseling, often focuses on the fear but, all too frequently, does not approach the "cure" or "recovery" with any concrete steps that will allow us to recognize our powerlessness over the crippling kind of fear. (Some fear is not debilitating and does not require the kind of recovery process contained in the 12 Steps. An appropriate fear of danger would be a good example. When I step on a poisonous snake, as I once did as a kid on a creek bank, I jump. Such a jump is a reaction to healthy, life-protecting fear.)

My problem with traditional one-on-one counseling is that it all too often fails to encourage an individual to move beyond the stumbling block of fear. My own experience with counseling was just that. Not only did several trained professionals fail to diagnose my problem, not one of them introduced me to a discipline through which I would discover the ultimate truth that God is the counselor and that God is powerless over nothing in my life. Nothing!

Am I opposed to traditional one-on-one counseling? Absolutely not! My point is simply this: counseling works best when it is grounded in the truth that it is God, or the Transcendent, or a Higher Power, who does the healing. I cannot heal anyone. I cannot even heal myself, but God can, and God is doing just that in my life, as well as in the lives of millions of recovering human beings, one day at a time.

Simple Steps...Costly Choices

The best of all worlds, from my perspective, is to enter into a counseling process, either one-on-one or as a couple with a counselor who will encourage and affirm your "outside" work in a recovery group. Well over 90 percent of the people I currently see are also working toward their own spiritual healing in the context of a 12 Step group. What is interesting, even fascinating, to me is that, like me, the vast majority of these folks are not now and have never been powerless over drugs or alcohol. But also like me, they have discovered that they are powerless over other forces or emotions, such as fear.

Paul Tillich writes of "the courage to be."[4] In my mind such courage is exactly what Step 8 entails. This Step is the courage to be reconciled if possible, but even more likely, it involves the courage to be peaceful. As you have, no doubt, decided or recognized in the course of working your own recovery program or in reading this book, inner peace requires courage. This is, I believe, what Tillich has in mind when he writes of "the courage to be."

According to Marsha Sinetar, Tillich means the following when he writes of courage: "the self-affirming life requires will: the will to have more life, to surpass ourselves. This sort of courage banishes everything cowardly; it is the opposite of submissiveness to external gods. Rather it affirms that which really is alive within, and is the will which compels the individual to take on the difficult, but perfectly natural life battles. It allows him to tackle the kind of small deaths which open him up to a larger life."[5]

Powerlessness over our fear is not a license for cowardice. This, to my mind, is Sinetar's point. Being caught in fear's grip is no reason for me to cower in some corner and refuse to live life to the fullest.

Step 8 is difficult. It requires that I take a hard look at how sick I am—so sick that I could hurt other people. Often such raw data is very unsettling. This knowledge does not square with how I see myself. Or, said another way, Step 8 is, in fact, quite difficult and not a little painful in that it requires that my old self "die" so that I might begin to live as a new being.

But before I can "die" to the old self as the initial step in gaining new life, I must first know as much as I possibly can about the old self. Therefore, it is incumbent upon me to fulfill the requirements of Step 8 with integrity, no matter how much pain this Step brings me.

Goethe writes, "And so long as you haven't experienced this: to die and grow, you are only a troubled guest on the dark earth." To me, what he is offering is the thought that until we are willing to die to our archaic allegiance to the image of ourselves as "right" and, therefore, "justified,"

Step 8: I prepare myself to make amends.

even in our brutality toward other human beings, we will continue to stumble about in this life in the shadows of our own unawareness and, therefore, will never discover peace.

The will to take on the difficult means abandoning our business-as-usual approach to life. It means giving up and turning over forever our familiar way of thinking and behaving. It further requires the willingness to face our fears, even when we have come to recognize that we are powerless over the very fears that Step 8 now compels us to face.

I believe that Step 8 is best worked in the context of solitude. One of my own aphorisms is "Sanity begins with solitude." Every day of my life, unless the weather is fiercely opposed to it, which is rare in Central Texas, I walk alone for one full hour. The first several minutes of that walk, I simply get into the awareness of how my body is moving and where the creaks and aches are presenting themselves to me for possible attention. Next I slip into a prayer, which invariably begins in the form of a petition for those who have injured me. Following that prayer of petition, I pray fervently for those whom I love, and for their continued healing and well-being. Eventually, I arrive at some concern for myself, and I work an 11th Step, which is simply asking God to empower me to do God's will. There is nothing elaborate about this habit. It is all very simple, but if I don't practice this discipline of "prayer walks," which are accomplished in the context of solitude, I will get "crazy" again very, very soon.

For me, sanity begins with solitude. I cannot imagine working this Step beyond the boundaries of solitude. It is, at times, so easy to become distracted, and the pain that Step 8 kicks up is so excruciating that it is tempting to distract myself with my daily regimen as opposed to probing my power to injure others.

Thomas Merton writes, "Man seeks unity because he is in the image of the One God. Unity implies solitude, and hence the need to be physically alone.[6] Many of us are afraid to be alone, however. I wrote this book in the cramped kitchen of a small rock cabin in the Hill Country; my only companion was a stray calico cat who wandered to my door each evening in hopes of receiving some kind of handout. I loved the solitude, but I did find myself strolling a couple of times a day to the pay telephone, where I could check in with the world I had abandoned a couple of weeks earlier.

As I mentioned in an earlier chapter, one of the countless gifts bestowed upon us by this program of spiritual healing is wisdom. And one truth that I have gleaned from this experience in working the Steps is the timeless truth that the only way out is through. Therefore, if you are a bit uneasy with solitude, I suspect it is because, deep down, you are frightened of being alone. Paul Tillich writes, "Loneliness can conquered only by those who can bear solitude. We have a natural desire for solitude because we are men. We want to feel what we are—namely, alone—not in pain and horror, but with joy and courage. There are many ways in which solitude can be sought and experienced."[7]

Tillich views solitude as the arena for the discovery of who we really are in the context of the struggle of both the forces of darkness and of light, which fight not only for our attention but also for our allegiance. Tillich continues:

> *So, first, this is what happens in our solitude: we meet ourselves, not as ourselves, but as the battlefield for creation and destruction, for God and the demons. Solitude is not easy. Who can bear it? It was not easy even for Jesus. We read—"He went up in the hills to pray. When evening came, he was there alone." When evening comes, loneliness becomes more lonely. We feel this when a day, or a period, or all the days of our life come to an end. Jesus went up to pray. Is this the way to transform loneliness into solitude and to bear solitude? It is not a simple question to answer.[8]*

Tillich is exactly right. The first thing that happens to us each and every time we deliberately seek solitude is that we do, indeed, meet ourselves, not as ourselves, but rather as the battlefield for creation and destruction, for God and the demons.

Therefore, obviously, solitude is never an easy enterprise, and the decision for solitude should never be made lightly. But in wrestling with your decision for solitude, keep this is mind: Solitude was also not easy even for Jesus and he willingly went before us into solitude in order to show us "the way."

In my view, this Step *must* be accomplished in solitude. There can be no other authentic route to working this Step. It is not the purpose of this Step, of course, to remain alone, isolated, and separated from our brothers and sisters, even from those we have injured. But the pain of this Step is so intense that it remains forever subject to distraction. Unless we make the courageous decision to accomplish Step 8 in solitude, I fear that it will never be accomplished.

The purpose of solitude is to send us back into the community, especially into the very core of our offense. Again, Tillich writes of the healing solitude engenders:

> *We have seen that we can never reach the innermost center of another being. We are always alone, each for himself. But we can reach it in a movement that rises first to God and then returns from Him to the other self. In this way man's aloneness is not removed, but taken*

Step 8: I prepare myself to make amends.

to the community with that in which the centers of all beings rest, and so into community with all of them. Even love is reborn in solitude. For only in solitude are those who are alone able to reach those from whom they are separated. Only the presence of the eternal can break through the walls that isolate the temporal from the temporal. One hour of solitude may bring us closer to those we love than many hours of communication....

It is the experience of being alone but not lonely, in view of the eternal presence that shines through the face of the Christ, and that includes everybody and everything from which we are separated. In the poverty of solitude all riches are present. Let us dare to have solitude—to face the eternal, to find others, to see ourselves.[9]

Step 8 is the "backing off" Step, which leads us inevitably to the goal of our spiritual evolution, that is, to be individual members of the same body we as Christians, in embracing Paul's theology, believe to be the body of Christ.

Scott Peck views God as the goal of our spiritual evolution.[10] This conviction is in no way meant to imply that we can be sovereign over and, therefore, in control of others. I have no problem in agreeing with Peck that God is the goal of the spiritual evolution we experience in the 12-Step recovery program. Further, I do not believe that it is too far-fetched for us to equate *being* in the body of Christ, or reconciled to one another, and "being God," as Peck puts it, as similar, if not the same thing. (This is the point that drives the so-called fundamentalists mad with Peck's *The Road Less Traveled*.)

Peck writes:

I have said that the ultimate goal of spiritual growth is for the individual to become as one with God. It is to know with God. Since the unconscious is God all along, we may further define the goal of spiritual growth to be the attainment of godhood by the conscious self. It is for the individual to become totally, wholly God. Does this mean that the goal is for the conscious to merge with unconsciousness so that all is unconsciousness? Hardly. We now come to the point of it all. The point is to become God while preserving consciousness. If the bud of consciousness that grows from the rhizome of the unconscious God can become itself God, then God will have assumed a new life form. ...We are born that we might become, as a conscious individual, a new life form in God.[11]

Throughout Christendom, folks croaked like a bullfrog, yipped louder than a kicked pup, and ran faster than a spooked rabbit when these words were first introduced to the culture back in the early 1980s. I even heard some mild repercussions in the urbane, congregation that I served at the time in Dallas. "This is new-age garbage!" I heard folks say. "Heresy!" someone else proclaimed beneath another tall steeple. But I've pondered this man's thinking off and on for the past fifteen years and I have come to the conclusion that what he writes above, specifically, God's being "the goal" of our own spiritual evolution, is twentieth-century language for precisely what Paul intended when he reminded the folks at Corinth of their true identity (1 Cor. 12:27): "Now you are the body of Christ and individually members of it."

Whether or not you concur that God is the goal of our spiritual evolution, I suspect that most of us will readily agree that Scott Peck is right when he writes about our avoidance of responsibility.[12] The fact is, we don't want the responsibility that attends any significant spiritual growth; therefore, we avoid it through all manner of psychological tricks, the most prevalent being denial. We in the church call ourselves the body of Christ while we fight regularly like a flock of buzzards over the same small scrap of road kill. We eschew reconciliation with about the same fervor that we avoid any serious commerce with solitude. Therefore, Step 8, if we are not very, very careful, can become no more substantive than one of those innocuous prayers of confession that I have mumbled for a lifetime in mainline church sanctuaries while my mind has remained consistently fixed on some issue far less costly.

In all the years I have served God through the traditional mainline church, I have not witnessed one person healed through any kind of traditional liturgy. Not one! In truth, we give little or no emphasis to healing at all. I suspect we're both embarrassed by the notion of "spiritual healing" and more than a little frightened of it. If someone were to experience such a miraculous healing, the truth is that we would feel great uneasiness. Officials at every level of any mainline ecclesiastical hierarchy might even brand a church that openly promoted healing as odd or even heretical. There might even be an investigation into what kind of theology was being practiced if folks began to experience all manner of healing in our mainline churches. Ultimately, any plethora of reported healing could even result in a pastor's being dismissed under a cloud of suspicion.

What fascinates me, however, on the occasion of the writing of this book, and following one year of service in what I would describe as a "noninstitutional" institution in which the senior pastor regularly proclaims publicly to a television audience of several million households that the 12 Steps are the Gospel "in drag," is that I have witnessed numerous "miracles" of healing.

Step 8: I prepare myself to make amends.

Is one church "better" than another? Of course not. To believe such nonsense is to miss the entire point. No, the point is that a church that openly promotes the 12 Steps is fostering healing while another church that reduces cathartic confessions to printed, "prefabricated" prayers of confession experiences very little, if any, real healing.

Effort is the key to Step 8. Healing requires that I put out the effort to face the loneliness of solitude so that I might get in touch, probably for the first time in my life, with the many ways I have injured others. The fact is that I don't want to do that. Further, I will go to just about any lengths to avoid doing Step 8, including, of course, finding myself a theology and a congregation in which such an earnest effort has been reduced, *unwittingly,* to the rote recitation of a generic confession that costs me little emotionally. Scott Peck terms this resistance "original sin":

> *So original sin does exist; it is our laziness. It is very real. It exists in each and every one of us—infants, children, adolescents, mature adults, the elderly; the wise or the stupid; the lame or the whole. Some of us may be less lazy than others, but we are all lazy to some extent. No matter how energetic, ambitious or even wise we may be, if we truly look into ourselves we will find laziness lurking at some level. It is the force of entropy within us, pushing us down and holding us back from our spiritual evolution.*[13]

Call it original sin, fear, stubbornness, denial, or whatever; the sad truth is this: I simply don't want to undertake any Step in which I must face my own ugliness. Like the rest of us human beings, I do not want to grow spiritually. Unless I accomplish this very difficult, and at times, unsettling Step, however, I will never experience any real peace. The unconscious will continue to gnaw at me with the painful reality of my own sins, and I will continue to languish in disquietude. Peace will never be mine.

Be that as it may, the honest fact is that, even knowing such to be true, I would still rather avoid the truth than stand face-to-face with myself and embrace the sordid facts regarding how it is that I have injured others. A big part of me longs to run as fast as I can from any such encounter, just as I once witnessed a man sprinting barefooted through the snow one morning more than two decades ago, when I was an intern minister in a small, loving congregation in Central Missouri.

During the night, a heavy snow had fallen. Because I inhabited a manse on the church property, I deemed it my responsibility to clear the church sidewalk and driveway of the new snowfall. While it was still dark I rolled out of bed quietly so as not to disturb my wife. I slipped my cold feet into the legs of a pair of warm, woolen trousers. I shuffled about in the darkness until I located enough warm clothing to protect me from the blizzard raging outside.

I waddled out of the front door, slipped a bit on the icy front porch, and very slowly made my way across a vacant lot buried in more than six inches of fresh snow. The church sanctuary remained unlocked, as always, and as I pulled open the front door, I bade good morning to the ghost I was convinced resided in the rafters of the ancient building and came to visit me regularly when I entered the sanctuary alone at night to practice my sermons.

I felt my way in the dark along the wall because I believed it to be far more convenient to locate the closet where the snow shovel was stored than to stumble in search of the light switch located on a distant wall.

With my fingers I traced the lines of the smooth, hundred-year-old paneling until I touched a small brass knob marking the entrance to a tiny storage closet. Very gently, like a robber cracking a safe, I turned the knob in a counterclockwise direction until I heard a distinctive click, signifying the opening of the closet door.

I pulled the door toward me and gently pushed my hand into the blackness of the closet in search of the smooth, worn handle of the snow shovel. Suddenly, I was aware that I was holding in the palm of my right hand what felt like a warm, partial sphere covered with a stubble reminiscent of my own face when I choose not to shave the whiskers on my neck beneath my beard.

This fellow whose chin I now held in my hand, whoever he was, appeared even more frightened than I. He shrieked as I screamed. He knocked me over in the dark as he scrambled to make an exit from the closet; as I lay on my stomach, I watched with a mixture of fear and fascination as the swinging door permitted me brief glimpses in the moonlight of his departure. This terrified man sprinted as fast as the fresh snow would permit on bare feet. He left his shoes at the church and, as far as I know, never returned for them.

What was his name? My intuition is that he carried most appropriately the moniker Everyman. His reaction was precisely my reaction when compelled to face the ugly truth that Step 8 specifically, and healing in general, requires that I face. Like the stranger in the moonlight, I would rather sprint across the snow-covered earth barefoot than stand face to face with my own sin.

Every instinct that aligns itself with the preservation of my elaborate system of denial kicks in when I am confronted with the information that Step 8 *requires* me to embrace as my truth. As long as I can run through the snow with the same wild, reckless abandon that I long ago witnessed

Step 8: I prepare myself to make amends.

on a winter morning in Missouri, I can put off for another moment, perhaps even several more hours or even days, the coming to the truth of my own sin. But as long as I run, I will find no peace. Peace lies only in stepping into my fear.

So, in working Step 8, keep the following foremost in your mind: this, like all 12 Steps, is not a Step of punishment or an attempt at humiliation. No, it is nothing less than a Step of love. For it is only through this listing of our injuries to others and through our ready willingness to make amends that we will discover love.

Thomas Merton writes of love more elegantly than anyone I read outside of the Scripture. He offers the following: "Love comes out of God and gathers us to God in order to pour itself back into God through all of us and bring us back to Him on the tide of His own infinite mercy."[14]

Step 8 is not about banishment and separation. It is about grace. It is not designed to punish or drown us in humiliation; rather, it is so structured, perhaps even ordained by God, to redeem us. Step 8 is not an invitation to shame, but a difficult Step toward what it means to experience salvation in this life.

D. H. Lawrence summarizes this Step more succinctly in the following poem than I could if I were to fill up several more pages:

Healing

I am not a mechanism, an assembly of various sections.
And it is not because the mechanism is working wrongly, that I am ill.
I am ill because of wounds to the soul, to the deep emotional self
and the wounds to the soul take a long, long time,
only time can help
and patience, and a certain difficult repentance,
long, difficult repentance, realization of life's mistakes and the freeing oneself
from the endless repetition of the mistake
which mankind at large has chosen to sanctify.

For more than twenty-five years I have enjoyed reading in a reference room in a seminary library where I am surrounded by journals, periodicals, and reference books pertaining to the Christian faith. The walls are decorated with Christian symbols and the names of the great reformers of the church are painted upon the wooden beams supporting the ceiling. It is a magnificent room, as cozy as my own den and yet challenging in that its spirit admonishes me in whispers and groans never to give up on the wonderful enterprise of discovering the secrets hidden in this room. For more than a quarter of a century I have visited this special room and within its four walls I have memorized both Greek and Hebrew vocabulary words and have written a play and numerous unread poems. I once also authored a Hebrew exegesis paper that surprised both the professor and me with its quality, and long ago, I pored over God only knows how many issues of *Sports Illustrated* in this room. It was in this place that I dared to dream, and I also listened carefully to the heartfelt yearnings of other students.

It is a wonderful, comfortable, and lovely room. One spring evening two years ago, I once again reclined in a comfortable chair in that splendid room and permitted my eyes to rest upon the beige plaster walls. Suddenly, to my surprise as well as to my joy, I discovered two figures that I had never before noticed. On the right side of the main entrance to the reference room at the top corner of the door's lintel, sits a stylized rendition of a serpent. And, of course, directly opposite that rendition sits a stylized version of a squatty little dove. Whoever had designed that room was intent upon sharing with those of us who would come to use it the Lord's admonition to be as harmless as a dove and wise as a serpent. Implicit in those symbols, of course, is Jesus' preface to the admonition: "Behold, I send you out amid wolves."[15]

In retrospect, I wish now that I had paid more attention to the symbols carved into the wall of my favorite room on earth. Though I heard the admonition often when I was a young seminarian, nothing could have prepared me for what I was to discover out there in the real world. Wolves inhabit the world, and all too often I fear that I have joined their vicious pack. It is this very viciousness in me that I come to face and then embrace as my personal truth in Step 8. If I am to experience any kind of genuine inner peace, I must make a list of those folks I have injured, and I must be willing to make amends to them all.

If I stop here in my program, I will never reach my goal of inner peace. And if I skip over this Step and Step 9 as well, my denial will come back to haunt me in the form of unconscious symbols, or symptoms. For me, that means depression and anxiety.

This is not a pretty Step, but it is, of course, an absolutely essential Step in our healing. It is simple to read the words of Step 8, but it is never easy to accomplish what they require of us. Be gentle with yourself. Recognize that God's power to forgive is more potent than even the sum total of our sins.

A good place to begin Step 8 is to go back to the preface of John's Gospel (John 1:5) and read these words: "The light shines in the darkness and the darkness has not overcome it."

Step 8: I prepare myself to make amends.

That also happens to be as good a place as any to conclude this chapter. God's blessing upon you as you step into solitude so that you may face yourself and discover God along the way.

References

[1] Truman Capote, *In Cold Blood* (New York: Random House, 1965), p. 340.
[2] Matt. 10:16 RSV.
[3] Marsha Sinetar, p. 14.
[4] Paul Tillich, p. 28.
[5] Marsha Sinetar, p. 15.
[6] Thomas Merton, *New Seeds of Contemplation*, p. 52.
[7] Paul Tillich, p. 21.
[8] Ibid., p. 23.
[9] Ibid., pp. 24–25.
[10] M. Scott Peck, *The Road Less Traveled*, p. 283.
[11] Ibid.
[12] Ibid., p. 301.
[13] Ibid., p. 273.
[14] Thomas Merton, *New Seeds of Contemplation*, p. 67.
[15] Matt. 10:16 RSV.

9

Blessed are the peacemakers, for they shall be called sons of God.

Matthew 5:9 RSV

Step 9: *I make direct amends to such people wherever possible, except when to do so would injure them or others.*

Will Campbell's one-sentence definition of Christianity is this: "We're all bastards, but God loves us anyway."[1] In all my rambling, listening, observing, and doing what little I could to make a contribution to the cause of God's kingdom, I've yet to bump into a better definition. "We are all bastards, but God loves us anyway." I like the definition. In fact, by the time any of us reach Step 9 in our program of recovery, the pretense, self-righteousness, and arrogance have all but been squeezed out of us, and we stand trembling before the throne of grace armed with little else but that one-sentence definition. To personalize it, I often confess the truth to God and even, on occasion, to a brother or sister. I boldly state, "I am a bastard, but God loves me anyway."

Part of what Step 9 is about is to recognize the truth of my identity. When I declare that I am a "bastard," which I hope you have deduced has nothing whatsoever to do with one's parentage, but, rather, is southern for "sinner," I am declaring the essence of my being. I am a sinner.

The truth is that I have injured many people in my close to fifty years upon this planet. As best I can figure it, I didn't intend to injure most of those folks, but I did injure them just the same. Others I sure did intend to injure. In fact, I went after them without thought to the consequences or even the slightest consideration of just how my personal declaration of "war" stacked up against what I professed to be my faith in Christ as the so-called Lord of my life. In a moment of passion, none of this made any real difference to me; I just went after folks.

Another spin on the word "bastard" in the culture that reared me is "hypocrite." I am a full-fledged hypocrite. In fact, I've seldom encountered anyone who was not, deep down, at some level of their being, living one way while their mouths professed a whole different "truth."

All of this is to demonstrate to the readers of this book that, as one of my seminary professors once wrote on a paper I had turned in to him, "You have a *firm* grip on the obvious." I wasn't bright enough or sufficiently erudite to decipher the full intent in that man's meaning, but in retrospect, I don't figure that the fellow was paying me much of a compliment. If he were to read what I have written as the opening for Step 9, he would no doubt feel compelled once again to write at the bottom of the page, just as he did a quarter of a century ago, "You have a firm grip on the obvious."

The fact is, I do. It has become painfully obvious to me that every one of us is a bastard, or a hypocrite, or, to employ a much more theologically erudite word, a sinner. I may, indeed, have a firm grasp upon the obvious, but so does a Swiss theologian whom that same seminary professor encouraged me to read as well as revere. Karl Barth offers in much more refined language a definition that is basically the same as Will Campbell's: "Man's becoming a law-breaker is the result of his fall from the covenant, of the disobedience with which he entered history and placed himself in the impossible situation of sin."[2]

Our powerlessness over sin has been our predicament from the very beginning in a Garden where one son murdered the other, where disobedience and its subsequent chaos reigned over a once-perfect order, and where rebellion hurled our spiritual ancestors toward eviction and certain misery. In my mind's eye, I can almost hear Adam whispering to Eve what I've heard folks offer in sighs almost too deep for words: "I wish we could return to the good old days."

This is the fundamental point of Step 9: there were no good old days. They never existed. They are nothing more than romanticized memories, a cultural myth. As I wrote in a previous chapter, our problem, as Paul so wisely informs us, lies not with our sins, but, rather, with our natural

Step 9: I make amends where possible.

proclivity for sin.

Step 9 is a step out of our sin and into what it means to crawl on our knees on the path of God's righteousness. It is my nature *not* to want to do that. It is my sinful, frightened nature to bury myself in a habit of denial and wrap myself in rationalizations as though they were a warm comforter offered me on a long winter's night.

Every time I even contemplate working this Step, I hear the voices in my head lulling me toward serious resistance with a siren song brimming with reasons why I don't really have to work Step 9. Some of those reasons sound a lot like this:

"I really didn't mean to."

"Keep in mind that what that other fellow did to me was far worse than what I did to him."

"After all, she started it!"

"She deserved it."

"Oh, now, she is just exaggerating."

"She wasn't really that hurt."

"Life ain't no church picnic."

"In reality, I did the woman a favor in teaching her to roll with the punches."

"Worse has certainly been done to me."

"It's a dog-eat-dog world."

"There is always grace, and besides, I know that God will forgive me whether or not I work Step 9."

And, perhaps, the most common as well as the most insidious:

"I'm too busy."

I'm a Civil War buff. And though I regard slavery as the most evil institution ever imposed upon any people, and though I marched for civil rights in the sixties, and though I attended for an academic year a predominantly black graduate school, I confess to being an inveterate student (as opposed to scholar) of the Confederacy.

In my mind, the greatest figure yet to walk upon this continent was none other than Gen. Robert E. Lee. It is not my purpose to praise this man, but I do admire him with close to the same reverence I give to biblical figures. Douglas Southall Freeman, in his definitive biography of Lee, tells of the great soldier's final surrender to U. S. Grant at Wilbur McClean's farmhouse in Appomatox Courthouse, Virginia. As General Lee approached that house for the purpose of surrendering the Army of Northern Virginia to Grant, he is reported by his biographer to have said (in paraphrase), "I would rather die a thousand deaths than to do what I am now called upon by duty to accomplish."[3]

Working Step 9 is not nearly so dramatic, of course, but believe me when I offer that I have experienced similar thoughts when I have walked into the life of someone I once injured for the express purpose of making an apology. I don't want to do it. If you have never done it, believe me when I tell you that it is anything but easy. To do Step 9, I must surrender any trace of pride and I must, necessarily, humble myself to the truth of my own sinful nature. But the good news underlying this very painful Step is that when I choose to make peace with a person I have hurt, I am also choosing to make peace with myself. Therefore, I can never have any real, lasting peace unless I first work this terribly difficult Step.

The way our personalities are constructed, interpersonal conflict is inevitable. And because all of us are sinners, it is also inevitable that we will end up injuring each other.

A young, gifted man in my life whom I will call Zack injured me deeply some time back. I had helped him enormously in the past, I thought. At one point, I had even served as his counselor and advocate. Months later, I discovered that for reasons that, I suspect, lay buried in his unconscious, this talented young man had both promoted and perpetuated very hurtful, and potentially damaging, rumors regarding my fitness as both a clergyman and a pastoral counselor.

Of course, not wishing to experience further injury, I withdrew from him immediately. Should I have confronted him? Possibly. But my decision about Zack is that he is not yet sufficiently in touch with his own shadow, to borrow from Jung, for me to be safe in any kind of genuine confrontation. This is precisely the principle to which I alluded in Chapter 7 regarding the wisdom of not subjecting oneself to further emotional abuse.

Zack has written me a couple of anguished letters about my withdrawal from him. He reports not to understand my decision for distance, since I had been both warm and supportive. What he failed to write to me was a request to come into my presence and work Step 9. If he had done that or were to do that today, I would gladly meet him, listen to his perception of how he injured me, and then give him a hug. Our relationship could be fully restored and, perhaps, strengthened.

Is my withdrawal a form of passive aggression? Is my intentional distance from him a socially acceptable, but subtle, way to injure him? Perhaps. I don't know for certain, but I have made a conscious decision to withdraw from the man for reasons having to do with self-protection, and, right or wrong, I have surrendered this decision to God.

Do I need to make the 9th Step to Zack? I have searched my heart and

Step 9: I make amends where possible.

soul on this one. I cannot figure out what I did to injure the man. There can be no doubt about one thing, though; today I am injuring Zack by withdrawing my affection from him. I am painfully conscious of that withdrawal, and I feel badly about it. But I am also conscious of being, in Jesus' words, a dove and, therefore, I do not speak ill of him.

As I write this book, I am somewhat satisfied, though not totally convinced, that my decision to "protect" myself from Zack through withdrawal is a sound, but imperfect, strategy. Perhaps someday he will seek to work Step 9, and at that time he will come to me and make amends for the hurt he has caused me. Once again, if such an opportunity ever presents itself, I will also be open to hearing from him how it is that I injured him.

I relate this personal slice of my pain to reiterate that maintaining functional human relationships is a very taxing and, at times, close to impossible task. There are occasions when you and I must play God in that we are called upon to make decisions that affect the lives of other human beings. And making the "right" or most ethical decision with a person like Zack was precisely one of those times for me. As long as I remain prayerful and uneasy with my decision, I will probably, though not certainly, remain on the right path.

Thomas Merton writes of the difficulty underlying all human commerce:

> *As long as we are on earth, the love that unites us will bring us suffering by our very contact with one another, because this love is the resetting of a Body of broken bones. Even saints cannot live with saints on this earth without some anguish, without some pain at the differences that come between them.*
>
> *There are two things which men can do about the pain of disunion with other men. They can love or they can hate.*
>
> *Hatred recoils from the sacrifice and the sorrow that are the price of this resetting bones. It refuses the pain of reunion . . .*
>
> *There is in every weak, lost and isolated member of the human race an agony of hatred born of his own helplessness, his own isolation. Hatred is the sign and the expression of loneliness, or of unworthiness or insufficiency. And in so far as each one of us is lonely, is unworthy, each one hates himself. Some of us are aware of this self-hatred, and because of it we reproach ourselves and punish ourselves needlessly. Punishment cannot cure the feeling that we are unworthy. There is nothing we can do about it as long as we feel that we are isolated, insufficient, helpless, alone. Others, who are less conscious of their own self-hatred, realize it in a different form by*

projecting it on to others. There is a proud and self-confident hate, strong and cruel which enjoys the pleasure of hating, for it is directed outward to the unworthiness of another. But this strong and happy hate does not realize that like all hate it destroys and consumes the self that hates, and not the object that is hated. Hate in any form is self destructive, and even when it triumphs physically it triumphs in its own physical ruin.

Strong hate, the hate that takes joy in hating, is strong because it does not believe itself to be unworthy and alone. It feels the support of a justifying God, an old idol of war, an avenging and destroying spirit. From such blood-drinking gods the human race was once liberated, with great toil and terrible sorrow, by the death of a God who delivered himself to the Cross and suffered the pathological cruelty of His own creatures out of pity for them.[4]

To work Step 9 means to become fully conscious. Hatred, incivility, and the dynamic of psychological projection, are all rooted in the fertile soil of the human unconscious. There is no doubt in my mind that the manner in which my young friend Zack "wronged" me is far more an expression of his unconscious than any kind of accurate report on either my ability or my character.

The same is, of course, true for me. The way I have wronged and injured others is far more an expression of my own unresolved unconscious conflicts than it is any kind of accurate portrayal of the individual on whom I have vented my wrath. Hatred, incivility, and projection are also the sins that keep me tied tightly to misery. To step out of this unconscious contract with misery, I must first, of course, become conscious. Therefore, as I stated above, Step 9 is a step out of the shadows of my unconscious war with myself and a step in the direction of healing and inner peace.

When I make this Step I would be wise to say to God and to myself something like the following prayer:

Lord, I have injured the person I am about to visit. I injured him or her because I, in truth, have never learned fully what it means to love me. And I go forth today to make an apology to this individual buttressed by the truth of your abiding grace and armed with the insight that life is seldom, if ever, fair. I go with no expectation of receiving warmth or enjoying hospitality. Neither do I step forward with even the remotest expectation of some kind of reciprocity, or quid pro quo arrangement between us. I go forward also with no expectation whatsoever for justice. In fact, I go with no expectation for anything except that in going my behavior might be pleasing to you, and that through

Step 9: I make amends where possible.

this difficult Step I might discover more of what it means to be peaceful. Please go with me so that I will be assured that in all that I do, I will remain an instrument of your peace.
Amen.

This is also a step in the direction of "personal power." But let us be clear about this. The power we discover in Step 9 can never be used to coerce or control another human being. That kind of power is political in nature. No, the power we discover in this Step is something far different from political power. This is the power to love, and this force we discover in ourselves through the working out of Step 9 is what can best be termed "spiritual power." And as Scott Peck writes, of the two, spiritual power and political power, the former is the most powerful in that it is through spiritual power that we "know with God."[5]

Years ago, I witnessed a man consciously trade his investment in political power for spiritual power. His was one of the most bizarre, and impressive, transformations I have ever seen. At the time I was waging war against a cadre of businessmen who were determined not to permit the municipal government to place a church-operated shelter for the homeless in close proximity to their neighborhood. The city fathers and mothers called a hearing, and I and the Episcopal priest I have mentioned previously in this book were invited to attend this hearing.

I had no argument to offer except that I had learned, even before I could read, the word "Inasmuch." "Inasmuch as you have done it to the least of these, my brethren, you have done it to me."[6] That was the sum of my evidence. I carried a briefcase with absolutely nothing in it because I figured that if I was going to my first-ever hearing, I should go armed with some kind of official symbol. That empty briefcase was my symbol.

As the priest and I entered the meeting room at city hall, I was immediately overwhelmed, and not a little frightened, by the crowd facing us. There were more than twenty-five of them and there were only two of us and my empty briefcase.

The second fact to register in my anxious awareness was that these prosperous-looking businessmen were being represented by an attorney, a kindly old gentleman whom I knew, and who had, since long before my birth, been a member of the same demonination that I now served as associate pastor. I recognized immediately that their choice of legal counsel was no coincidence.

The old gentleman smiled at me, and I nodded in silent response at the obvious arrangement now before me. I wondered to myself about this man's level of comfort with the side he had chosen, or that, more likely, had chosen him. Suddenly, my empty briefcase felt more worthless than ever.

The meeting began poorly. One of the prosperous men, dressed in what I judged to be a thousand-dollar pin-striped suit, leaned across the table from me and said, "Dr. Lively, the Bible teaches that God helps those who help themselves."

I simply could not restrain myself. I turned to this well-groomed young businessman and answered, wearing a smile of new found confidence: "That is not in the Bible, sir. It is to be found in *Poor Richard's Almanac*. Its author is Benjamin Franklin, and the last time I checked, no one in the church has yet to canonize either that brilliant, but lusty, old patriot or his writings." And then my own surliness showed its ugly face as I continued: "Please don't quote the Scripture to me, sir, unless you know it."

My priest friend kicked my ankle hard. The room was brimming with ego, the battle was on, and discord was swirling about in the currents of a power that was anything but spiritual.

At that point in the meeting a man I later learned had made his millions peddling all kinds of nuts to the well-heeled citizens of our city could scarcely contain his rage. He half climbed upon the table and began an exaggerated crawl in my direction as if he had been suddenly transformed into some mythic, obscene dragon. The more genteel gentleman who had moments before confused Poor Richard with Holy Writ, grabbed the man by his ankles as he made his half-hearted lunge at me across the table.

Feeling the "friendly" restraint offered by his confederate, this red-faced man now barked at me this question: "Why don't you just take these bums into your own church and get the hell out of our neighborhood?"

I smiled, and said, "We do. We've been doing just that for years. There is just not enough room."

The man was far from finished. "Well, son, you could put them all in your damn sanctuary. There should be sufficient room there for all the bums and winos in this town."

I heard his friends laugh as I studied the now-sad face of the old man this rowdy group had selected for their legal counsel.

I answered: "That is not a bad idea. How about you coming over and joining our church to help me convince the folks who govern the place to let us do just that?"

A second whack on the ankle with the toe of a boot. I flinched, gripping my new, empty briefcase.

The attorney rose from his chair. He lifted his briefcase, which was, I

Step 9: I make amends where possible.

suspect, far from empty, and paused to collect his thoughts as a hush fell over the hearing room. He gazed at me with his eyes filled more with sorrow, I thought, than with any other emotion, and offered in a low monotone, "I quit. You men can work this out on your own, but I will not represent anyone who fights against Jesus. I quit. Take your fee and give it to some other lawyer. The woods are full of young Turks who are more than a little ready to take your money."

He turned and walked out of the room, and in that wonderful moment I witnessed for the first time in my life the clear delineation between political power and spiritual power.

Scott Peck is right; of the two, spiritual power is by far the stronger. And it is precisely this sense of spiritual power (vis-à-vis political power) with which I arm myself when I move forward to Step 9.

Political power, at its best, seeks compromise; at its worst, it chases vengeance. Spiritual power, however, longs for only one thing—love. Therefore, when I choose to work Step 9, I do so in the context of a love that bids me to make peace wherever possible, unless to do so would inflict even further injury.

Ten years ago, I wrote articles, stories, and anecdotes for a marvelous little magazine known as *The Other Side*. Some months ago, I was thumbing through the pages of a complimentary copy I once received as part of my writing contract with those radical (meaning rooted in the Word of God) Christians. And it was on those slick pages that I happened upon a story that stunned me. In fact, this story stirred me so much that, following a careful reading, I stood up and went for one of my daily long walks in the cause of digesting the miracle I had encountered.

This article "remembered" the Kent State killings on that infamous day in May 1970. I was in my first year of seminary when the tragic news was broadcast to us via television that students whose only crime had been to protest the war in Vietnam had been shot to death on the campus of one of this nation's universities. These children had been fired upon by a unit of National Guardsmen who had sworn an oath to keep the peace on that campus. And in those terrible days of tension and heartache, what it meant to "keep the peace" had obviously come to mean, at least in the minds of the men who fired their weapons, the heinous act of murder.

I remembered the day all too well as I read the article in *The Other Side*. I recalled where I was standing on the seminary campus when a fellow student ran to my place on the sidewalk to inform me that students at Kent State University had been murdered for exercising rights guaranteed by the First Amendment.

I remembered fighting the tears as I made my way to the small apartment my wife and I inhabited, and I recalled sitting before the tiny screen of our portable television deep into the night posing to myself, to my wife, and to God questions for which there were no answers.

Yes, I remembered it all, and then I turned a page of *The Other Side* to discover a list of National Guardsmen who had agreed to offer a public, written apology to the families and friends of those who had been slain. These men offered no excuse, no rationalization, but simply an apology for the sin they had committed. These soldiers had returned to the scene of their crime to make peace, and in a very real sense they had come, whether they labeled it as such or not, to take Step 9 on the road to spiritual maturity and the inner peace it promises.

Their sense of power had shifted dramatically from political to spiritual, and their act of courage affected me dramatically; I suspect it had a similar impact on everyone who read their official written apology.[7]

Political power strangles human relationships with the choke hold of coercion; spiritual power liberates us to love enough so that we might make peace, even with, most especially with, those we once regarded as enemies.

Since I first read it, I have been deeply touched by a poem written by Antonio Machado entitled "The Wind, One Brilliant Day." In this work he paints with words a magnificent picture of a man who confesses to himself, and I suppose to God, that, by his own fumbling, he has destroyed a precious garden once entrusted to him. In what was once a beautiful garden, the flowers have died and their fragrance has vanished on some long-forgotten breeze.

My response to the poet prior to my discovery of these 12 Steps is that I had strangled the very garden that was once vouchsafed to me by love. In fact, I damn near choked it to death with my adamant insistence upon the use of the brute force of political power, which for the first four decades of my life I, unfortunately, confused with what it means to love. I invested forty years in strangling myself, regularly choking those I professed to love, and calling such abuse, manipulation, and insanity, love.

As I have come to see it, Step 9 is the living out and, therefore, the full proclamation of what it means to be spiritually powerful. The paradox of it all is that when I willingly decide to make myself vulnerable is when I am at my very strongest. I've always had it backwards. For years I believed that I was at my peak when I showed no one even a hint of rust, much less a full chink in what I regarded as my shiny defenses.

The theologian I have cited so often, Dietrich Bonhoeffer, claims that it is our work to prepare for the coming of Christ in the world.[8] After having

Step 9: I make amends where possible.

worked these Steps in the context of the recognition of my own sinful nature, I have come to believe that Step 9 does precisely what Bonhoeffer describes: it proclaims the coming of grace to a sad, dark, tired world.

In every sense of the word, Step 9, then, is a step of repentance. As before in Chapter 5, Paul Tillich describes that mysterious moment in our lives when we make conscious connection with the truth that this decision for repentance, and for the bringing to fruition of our spiritual power, is God's work:

> *But in some moment He [God] appears as God. The unknown force in us that caused our restlessness becomes manifest as the God in Whose hands we are, Who is our ultimate threat and our ultimate refuge. In such moments it is as though we were arrested in our hidden flight. But it is not an arrest by brute force, but one that has the character of a question. And we remain free to continue our flight. This is what happened to the disciples: they were powerfully arrested when Jesus first called them, but they remained free to flee again. And they did when the moment of trial arrived.*[9]

Any attempt at serious repentance involves the full recognition that our hands are God's hands, and such a responsibility invariably brings with it fear.

Ultimately, Step 9 calls us to accept responsibility for our sins and to express our deep sense of remorse to those we have injured except where to do so would cause further harm. This is an awesome responsibility, and one that can never be taken lightly. It is Step 9 that, in the words of Bonhoeffer, "prepares the way for the coming of grace" and, for me, is, at the same time, the most terrifying of all 12 Steps.

And the truth is that the frightened part of me wishes to dodge the responsibility of it all. Ever since I first read the closing verse of Edwin Arlington Robinson's classic poem "Miniver Cheevy," I have identified with the deep pain it expresses with such cryptic, almost brutal insight into what it means to avoid:

> Miniver Cheevy, born too late,
> Scratched his head and kept on thinking;
> Miniver coughed, and called it fate,
> And kept on drinking.

Responsibility is as frightening as it is treacherous. Gerald May writes regarding the difficulty of accepting responsibility: "God, in whose image we are made, instills in us the capacity for relentless tenacity, an assertiveness that complements our yearning hunger for God. But most of us overdo it; our spirit of assertiveness quickly becomes the spirit of pride."[10] Step 9 is not a step into pride; rather, it is a conscious step out of my unconscious defenses, pride being but one among several. More, it is a Step into the paradox of making myself powerful through the act of willing, conscious vulnerability.

Years ago I stopped at a small Protestant church in the Midwest and heard a man preach whom I had heard judged rather harshly, as well as regularly, by his colleagues to be stiff, stilted, and more than a little boring. My motives were anything but pure in halting on my journey to some other place to hear this preacher. Years before I had been offered this very pulpit, but for more reasons than I have space remaining in this chapter, I decided against accepting the invitation to become the pastor of this historic, dying church.

On this particular summer morning the sanctuary was less than half full. I slipped into the back pew, hoping, of course, not to be recognized by the folks whom I had long ago turned down.

As the man walked into the pulpit of the splendid sanctuary, I was impressed by both his youthfulness and the fatigue and sadness etched into his countenance. I immediately congratulated myself on having made the "correct" decision.

As he began to preach, I expected the worst, but what the sad man offered was nothing less than the most honest description of his own anguished childhood with a mother who abandoned him to a rather hapless father so that she might spend what remained of her life chasing dreams lying at the bottom of a bottle. His sermon was more of a personal testimony of one man's tortured childhood than it was any kind of well-crafted exegetical expression of some piece of Scripture. Immediately I wondered what had brought him to such a catharsis in the presence of folks I knew from my own experience to be pretty rough customers.

He wrapped up his final point with tears welling in his eyes. It was one of the most powerful experiences of my life because I witnessed in this young, obviously frightened, preacher the willingness to make himself vulnerable. He sought neither pity nor any kind of empathy or connection with his pain. Neither did he whine or perceive of himself as stuck in some self-denigrating cycle. No, he simply made himself vulnerable, and in that conscious act of boldness, he demonstrated to me, and to every man, woman, and child in the pews, I suspect, a humility that serves as the bedrock for all that it can possibly mean to be spiritually mature. In a word, the man was "powerful."

I lingered in the narthex of the church so that I might shake his hand following the worship service. During those several minutes I was moved

Step 9: I make amends where possible.

by how the people of his congregation lined up to offer a sincere word of gratitude. I suspect that he had touched them in ways for which there are no words to describe the mystery of the experience. And as I stood observing him, I wondered how he had gained a reputation for being drier than West Texas in summer.

Years later I heard that this man had been "run off" by this very same congregation. What was their complaint? He was boring, they charged. Nothing more than that. I can't begin to speculate about the political machinations of that situation, but on the Sunday morning I sat at the man's feet, I was anything but bored. I was, in my view, in the presence of a man who was so powerful as to be mesmerizing in that he willingly chose to make himself exceedingly vulnerable to any who were willing to listen. There was not even a shred of false pride in what that man had to say. Nothing spilled from his mouth but the power born of integrity.

You see, there can be no place whatsoever for pride in the context of what it means to be spiritual, or to seek spiritual maturity. Most people, I believe, long for political power, but there are precious few among us, like the young man I once heard preach, who are willing to do what is required to live a life dedicated to the truth as they perceive it. These are the spiritually mature among us, and their power lies in their willingness to swap false pride for a conscious vulnerability.

Such people muster the courage to take Step 9. And make no mistake about it, Step 9, like the Steps that precede it, requires enormous moral courage.

Some years ago, a man I knew quite well in a social context visited my office for the express purpose of asking me to listen to his dilemma. As he sat in the rocking chair I was mighty fond of at the time, he began to rock rather frenetically, and then he just blurted out as beads of perspiration dotted his brow: "I've had an affair!"

It was not, of course, the first time I had ever heard such words. I sat in silence as I waited to see what this man wanted from me regarding the problem of his affair.

"I feel so ashamed. I am daily flooded with guilt. I can't sleep at night. I don't go to church anymore. I'm racked with turmoil, and I very much want to confess this thing to my wife and get it off my chest."

I waited for grace to take its course in this man's thinking. A protracted silence ensued, and finally I asked, "Where are you right now in the relationship with the other woman?"

His answered surprised me some. "I haven't seen her in more than 10 years. We both broke it off simultaneously. We realized at about the same time that it was not good for either one of us. It was more an 'affair of the heart' than anything physical, but it was an affair."

I admired his courage as well as his willingness to make himself vulnerable to me through his dedication to the truth. I asked, "What good could it possibly do your wife to know this now? It would only hurt her, is my guess."

The man wagged his head in the direction of "No!" obviously unmoved by my words.

"Look," I said, "you tell me that it is over. Right?"

"Right," he answered, without glancing up at me.

"Do you believe that God has forgiven you?"

"I do," he professed without hesitation. "At least I do believe that!"

"And the former 'affair' is not impinging, then, on your life or upon your wife's life or upon your marriage, is it?"

"No, it's entirely over. I will never see the woman again. I wish her only the best, but she and I will never enjoy any kind of relationship again, not even a letter or a postcard. Nothing!"

"Well, then, it strikes me," I continued, "that for you to tell your wife now would be to injure her."

The man jumped to his feet, stared straight into my eyes, and exclaimed "Really?!"

"Really."

As he shook my hand vigorously he offered, "You're the best damn counselor in this whole city."

Of course, we both recognized immediately that his enthusiastic characterization of me was as far-fetched in the direction of positive exaggeration as the one Zack had offered in the opposite direction. But in my mind the truth was that by making an apology to his wife regarding something she did not need to know, and by refusing to harm her with information that was in no way impinging upon her present life, this man was unwittingly working Step 9.

Now wait just a minute, you may say. Did I not spend the first several chapters of this book building a mighty strong case for rigorous honesty? I did, in fact, do just that. There can be no doubt about it, and I stand by what I wrote. But you see, the criterion for making a decision to share painful information in the context of Step 9 is this: if the circumstances no longer affect a person's life, and if an innocent person I love would be injured by no longer relevant information, there is, in my mind, no sound, or even ethical, reason to injure that person with that information. As my granddaddy used to say, "Water under the bridge can't flood upstream."

This is not a license to lie. Had the man told me he was currently

Step 9: I make amends where possible.

involved in an affair, I would have invited, even encouraged, him to share the information immediately with his wife. She would deserve the truth because his deceit was affecting her life. If he wanted to redeem the relationship, truth was his only hope. But the illicit relationship was over and, by God's grace, this tortured man had terminated all contact with the woman and she with him. It had been years since he had seen her, and he, through the process of entering and then ending this relationship, had learned a good bit about himself and about his own capacity for sin. In my view, his guilt seemed to be punishment enough.

The man's problem was guilt, not deceit. There is a marked difference between the two. Deceit requires honesty, while in the context of guilt, or remorse, discretion may well be a far more redemptive alternative.

I offer this anecdote to remind us that this Step is in no way to be perceived as a license for brutality. Brutality, or telling all that we know, is overkill and may even reach the point of emotional violence. There is no place whatsoever for violence in recovery or in our quest for spiritual maturity. Keep in mind that Step 9 states that we should make amends *except* where to do so would cause further injury. Once again, I am faced with a decision, and one more time on this path to inner peace I am mandated to "play God." Such is simply a part of the cost of health. No decision on this path should ever be made without our first surrendering it to the will and wisdom of God, who is the wellspring of all real joy in this life.

Step 9 is terribly difficult, and on the surface appears to be anything *but* a joyful experience. The way I view it, Step 9 is that gentle bend in the road on this arduous journey during which, for the very first time, real joy comes into sight and leads me to hope that happiness is something more than an ephemeral illusion.

In my experience, Step 9 portends joy in the manner that thunder heralds life-sustaining showers. Be on the lookout for joy. It comes with healing, and this kind of joy is authentic and may be trusted. In my view it arrives for one reason—to encourage us on our path toward God.

References

[1] Campbell, *Brother to a Dragonfly*, p. 221.

[2] Karl Barth, *The Heidelberg Catechism for Today* (Richmond: John Knox Press, 1964), p. 37.

[3] Douglas Southall Freeman, *R. E. Lee: A Biography*, vol. 4 (New York: Charles Scribner's Sons, 1935), p. 120.

[4] Thomas Merton, *New Seeds of Contemplation*, p. 72.

[5] M. Scott Peck, *The Road Less Traveled*, p. 286.

[6] Matt. 25:40 RSV.

[7] Lesley Wischman, "With Mercy and Sorrow," *The Other Side Magazine* (May–June 1990), pp. 34–37.

[8] Dietrich Bonhoeffer, *Ethics* (New York: Macmillan, 1949), p. 137.

[9] Paul Tillich, p. 103.

[10] Gerald May, p. 19.

10

Do not be conformed to this world but be transformed by the renewal of your mind, that you may prove what is the will of God, what is good and acceptable and perfect.

Romans 12:2 RSV

Step 10: *I continue to take personal inventory and when I am wrong, I promptly admit it.*

When I was sixteen years old, I did my best to convince old Pancho to go squirrel hunting with me over in the woods beyond the first cow pasture. It was a marvelous November morning, as crisp as it was bright. And Pancho was regarded, at least by my kin, as the finest squirrel dog in the whole of Houston County, Texas. The dog declined my invitation and turned his head away from my pleadings, as he lay in the cold shadows of the house's foundation.

Granddaddy would take Pancho to the woods regularly and plop himself down on the smooth surface of a fat hickory stump and whittle until the dog began an incessant barking. Pancho did all the work. He could sniff a squirrel in a tree quicker than a skunk can spray stink. Granddaddy would amble over to the tree where Pancho was barking, and he would hush old Pancho with one sweep of his arm in the air. With that silent signal, our black and white border collie would whine, moan some, and dance about in circles as his master studied the situation.

Granddaddy would begin "visiting" with that old boar squirrel. He would scrape the rough bark of the tree's trunk with a twig he had been whittling on and he would chirp and bark and sound more like a squirrel than even a squirrel can. Pancho would remain agitated, but he would more or less maintain his own counsel as Granddaddy visited with that squirrel.

Soon enough, the boar squirrel would grow curious enough to peek out over the branch, and that would be his biggest, not to mention his last, mistake. Granddaddy would fire his rifle, and we would enjoy fried squirrel with all the trimmings for supper. (In East Texas, dinner is the noon meal.) Now if you can't appreciate how tasty that supper was, then I know your roots are not in the country. That's okay; you're invited to read on anyway.

So you can see my dilemma right off. I needed Pancho if my hunt was to prove successful. I had invested a full year in junior high school teaching myself how to bark like a squirrel and, in my mind, the time had arrived to test my skill in the context of dumbfounding sure-enough East Texas red squirrels.

More times than I can recall, I have visited with Colorado squirrels and Missouri squirrels, and have even talked a few pretty cagey Arkansas Ozark squirrels out of their nests, but I never did shoot at any of them. Today I am satisfied that an East Texas red squirrel is the brightest four-legged creature on Earth. As folks say in that part of the country, I'm mighty proud (meaning glad) that old Noah thought to invite a pair of red squirrels to climb aboard the ark. Had he omitted such an invitation, the rich culture of East Texas would have been diminished significantly.

Old Pancho remained recalcitrant, though. No kind of verbal inducements could coax him to abandon the security of the foundation shadows. He and I both owned the same truth: I was not my granddaddy, and when it came to hunting, old Pancho was a one-man dog.

I slipped into the house unnoticed and lifted a pork rib from Grandmother's platter in the center of the antebellum dining room table. I tucked that purloined rib into the right rear pocket of my blue jeans. Within minutes I was back in Pancho's face, begging, but this time also brandishing a plump pork rib.

Once again Pancho refused, but I sensed that now I had piqued his interest. I tied the pork rib to the frayed end of some fishing twine and hurled it beneath the foundation. Pancho bit harder than a trophy bass, and I yanked it out of his mouth. He rolled out from beneath that foundation, chasing the pork rib that I twitched on the end of the fishing twine.

We made an odd pair, old Pancho and I, as we crossed the sand hill on

Step 10: I continue to work on being truthful.

our way to the back woods. I marched with my rifle hoisted to my right shoulder, and old Pancho danced frenetically in close circles as he whined, moaned, barked, and sniffed the right rear pocket of my jeans, where I had hidden the rib.

Once we reached the woods, I sat upon the same stump my granddaddy used for whittling. Pancho flat refused to hunt. He danced and whined some more, and then dropped his plump body to the thick carpet of fallen leaves and watched me sit and stare back at him. I tried reasoning with that dog, but I learned that you can never reason with any creature, human or otherwise, that has made up its mind. The obvious fact was that old Pancho had definitely reached his own conclusion about this adventure: he was not about to hunt.

I extracted the pork rib from my pocket and tossed it toward Pancho. He immediately dug it out of the dirt like a right fielder on his way to the Hall of Fame, and he never bothered to offer so much as a glance of gratitude. He turned and galloped back to the shadows, where he invested the remainder of the weekend alternately gnawing on the pork rib and napping. I never *could* convince that dog to hunt.

For many of us, even those of us who are in recovery, our behavior is a lot like old Pancho's. We avoid adventures that may bring us great joy by choosing to remain stuck in the shadows of our own foundations.

Step 10 is the step into the light. The light is truth, and truth is the light. That is the biblical witness. And the Gospel of John (1:5) informs us in its preface that "the light shines in the darkness and the darkness has not overcome it." The darkness is our fear, and the shadows in our lives are the lies we tell ourselves and others in a vain attempt to keep ourselves "safe." The very simple reason any of us lie is because, for whatever reason, we have become afraid, even terrified, of the truth. Over time, lying can become a habit, and even a very significant, not to mention, destructive facet of our disease. Therefore, it is the purpose of Step 10 to keep us in the light by keeping us grounded in the truth.

Recently I was ten minutes late to a meeting. As I drove up to the radio station where I was scheduled to tape a practice interview with a guest on a proposed talk show, I immediately launched into a strategy. "Now what shall I tell my friends? What excuse shall I offer? Better yet, what exciting story can I fabricate to make my life sound even more fascinating than it actually is. I might as well impress these people if I'm going to the trouble to lie to them."

Then Step 10 clicked in, and I thanked God both for the Step and for the awareness it brings. I parked my pickup, climbed out of the cab, sauntered into that radio station, greeted my friends, and said, "I am sorry that I am late. I have no excuse. I am just plain ol' late."

I have to practice Step 10 several times a day, because the disease has created in me one artful, highly skilled, in fact, quite credible liar. The great majority of my lies over the years have been "harmless," but that very belief, which has served as my primary rationalization, is itself a great lie.

There are no harmless lies. If they are lies, they are not harmless, because, invariably, all lies injure us. They keep us sick and stuck in our disease, even if they do not directly or dramatically affect anyone else's life. Any power that keeps me sick is far from harmless.

To stay on the path of recovery, I *must* therefore remain dedicated to living an honest life every minute of every day, for as soon as I begin my rationalization of the "harmless lies syndrome," I'm on the road once again to slipping. Remember that frequent slips often lead to the kind of falls that don't stop until, once again, we have hit bottom.

Frederich Beuchner offers that "we are as sick as our secrets," and about that I believe that he is exactly right.[1] Step 10 is the conscious Step we take so that we might commit ourselves, once and for all, to reporting the truth, even when, and especially when, a lie would be much easier, more fun, and certainly far more convenient.

Every time I lie, I capitulate to fear. Every time I face my fear, even the fear of offering a necessary confrontation to someone I love or to someone I fear, I take a small step in the direction of recovery and toward what it means to be spiritually mature.

Dr. Gerald Mann, who is the senior pastor of the church—actually I call it a "miracle" more than a church—where I currently serve as a teacher and counselor in residence, is a gifted storyteller. He is also a healthy man and, therefore, he is a truth teller. I enjoy very much this man's unique gift for storytelling, both in and beyond the four walls of the Riverbend Church's worship center.

When he is on the threshold of an embellishment, he offers the following disclaimer: "Now there is some hair on this story." Such is his way of saying, "Hey, this story is embellished, but sit back and enjoy it anyway." There is no harm, then, in the story, because we all know it to be pumped up with a little air so as to heighten the message.

If we continue to lie without offering such disclaimers, and without stopping long enough to differentiate our exaggerations from the truth, we will only continue to make ourselves sick. I believe that Beuchner is exactly right: we will become as sick as our secrets.

Therefore, if we choose to work the 12 Steps of Recovery, we can no longer harbor secrets from those we trust, from God, or even from our-

Step 10: I continue to work on being truthful.

selves. In effect, that is precisely what denial is: a secret we attempt to hide from God, others, and even from ourselves. Denial, then, invariably and over time, makes us very sick.

A young graduate student visited my office more than a decade ago in Dallas. I'll call him Jerry. Prior to beginning his search for healing, every week of his adult life, he purchased a condom at the local drugstore and then prowled for a prostitute until he found some woman who was willing to "service" him, as opposed to love him, for what meager fee his graduate student budget might permit.

When we first began our work together, he failed to mention his weekly forays into the red light district of Dallas. Instead, he moaned some about all manner of disjointed, amorphous complaints having to do with his mother, father, professors, ex-girlfriends, and even God.

I found myself becoming increasingly bored, and I even came to dread our weekly visits. Boredom for a counselor usually points to one thing: the client is not "into" any authentic issue. More to the point, the client is not telling the truth, or all the client is offering the therapist is a veil of denial. Denial breeds boredom in the counseling office much like a skunk kicks up panic at a picnic. It's pretty close to axiomatic.

On his next visit, I confronted Jerry early in the session. Tears welled in his eyes, and he confessed that once in New York City he had run up a tab of more than three thousand dollars in one evening on his wealthy grandfather's credit card by paying women to table dance. According to Jerry, the saying in the business is "the bigger the bill the greater the thrill." I don't know how much thrill my young client Jerry got out of that evening in New York, but he did walk away with one enormous bill that he was later compelled to explain to his grandfather.

Only because I dreaded my own boredom, I confronted Jerry with these words: "Jerry, I have something to share with you. Actually, it's a confrontation, of sorts. No, that is not right. It is not a confrontation of sorts, it is a confrontation. I have come to believe that you're a sex addict."

Within days following that painful, poignant moment in our work together, he began a recovery program with a fervor that I have rarely witnessed in any client. Today he is a highly respected professional practicing his specialized craft on the West Coast and, by God's grace, he reports to me that he is now happily married and remaining sober, or "straight" as he terms it, one day at a time.

Denial is lying. It is nothing less and nothing more than that. It is just plain old garden-variety, ordinary lying. And lying is invariably a reaction to fear. If fear is the core of the disease, and I remain convinced that it is, then to lie is simply to collude with the disease. It is the worst possible decision I can make if I become dedicated to the kind of genuine healing that leads to spiritual maturity and its gift of inner peace.

If I want to put a campfire out, I would be plain stupid to pour kerosene on the embers. The same is true, of course, for this disease. Every time I lie, I am pouring kerosene onto smoldering embers. I am encouraging the disease's presence in my life, and welcoming its destructive forces into my soul, where they may in time, and with my full permission, ravage me.

Step 10 is the Step of prevention and maintenance. It is the Step that keeps me out of the shadows and holds me in the full light of my abiding faith in God. For me to remain on the path to healing, I *must* cultivate that faith daily.

If I discount my faith, or the whole of the biblical witness, as nothing more than one more fairy tale or a mere illusion, I will likely remain quite vulnerable to the very fear that so yearns to drag me back into its clutches. A steadfast faith in one higher than myself is the anchor that binds me to the truth and it is the only avenue any of us in recovery have yet discovered out of the shadow. Therefore, cultivation of the faith through such rigorous and daily disciplines as prayer, contemplation, Bible study, confession, and corporate worship is *essential* to keeping us in the light of truth.

If I go about this life making up my own "truths," quite soon I will be almost hopelessly lost. It is true enough that all truth is discovered, but the bedrock principle underlying that modern proverb is that there is a truth to be discovered. Truth, then, if it is truth, is discovered and never concocted.

God is the truth. It is my work, as well as each person's life task, to discover God and to discover who God is for each individual. The God I discover will quite likely not be the God you discover. What God wants of me and requires of me will not be what God wants and requires of anyone else.

But even in the wake of such perceived differences, God remains truth. Therefore, I must speak the truth and live the truth in order to remain close to God. The irony in all of this for me is that I don't know a whole lot more to write about God except to say that God is the truth.

Therefore, when I am late to an appointment and I lie regarding the reasons, I am distancing myself from God. When I tell myself and others that I don't have to follow the rules of this life that govern the behavior of others, I am also distancing myself from God. When I whisper into my own ear that I am so very, very special that I can be the god of my own life or can replace God with all manner of false idols, I am, once again,

Step 10: I continue to work on being truthful.

distancing myself from God.

Every decision I make concerning telling the truth every day of my life either brings me closer to or takes me farther away from God. If I make lies a daily practice, that is, if I make it my habit to capitulate to my fear, I will continue to distance myself from God. The farther I remove myself from my daily truths, and the farther I distance myself from God, the more ill I will surely become. It is just that simple.

Thomas Merton writes:

> *How many people there are in the world today who have "lost their faith" along with the vain hopes and illusions of their childhood. What they called "faith" was just one among all other illusions. They placed all their hope in a certain sense of spiritual peace, of comfort, of interior equilibrium, of self-respect. Then when they began to struggle with the real difficulties and burdens of mature life, when they became aware of their own weakness, they lost their peace, they let go of their precious self-respect, and it became impossible for them to "believe." That is to say it became impossible for them to comfort themselves, to reassure themselves, with the images and concepts that they found reassuring in childhood.*[2]

Inner peace specifically and recovery in general require what I term the appropriation of an "adult God" on the part of the individual seeking recovery and inner peace. This does not mean that God has grown up; rather, the term implies the necessity of developing a personal image of God that can withstand the chronic challenges, temptations, and vicissitudes of our hectic lives in this adult world. More succinctly, the god of my childhood can no longer serve me.

As I have mentioned, I went to college once and to seminary twice. The first time I attended seminary, I remained for three years; the second time I attended classes and authored papers over a period of four years on a part-time basis. All of this is to say that I have spent no small amount of time investigating God for myself. The God of my childhood and the strict, stern God of my days of compulsory chapel at a small liberal arts college in Sherman, Texas, is not the same God to whom I pray and upon whom I rely today. The God of my days of seminary training is not big enough to guide me as I approach my fiftieth birthday.

Of course, God has not changed. I have. I have grown, and the very best news that I can report to anyone about myself is that I am still growing. But the one constant throughout the whole of my life is this: no matter what I learn or unlearn, decide or redecide, commit to or abandon, God remains the truth.

The personal, emotional connection I have made to the truth of God since I began my own discipline of recovery and spiritual growth is what sustains me on a daily basis. As long as I speak and live the truth, I feel the sustenance that comes from being aligned with the truth. However, the minute I begin to veer—that is, fail to speak, as well as live, the truth—I begin to feel separated from that sustenance. I have learned the hard way that my sustenance has never abandoned me. No, it is I who have abandoned it the minute I begin a trip on this trail of lies.

In many of my anecdotes, especially those involving clients or friends, I have changed the names and falsified the details to protect the anonymity of the people involved. I made this decision as a conscious act and as an acceptable, not to mention wise, practice in the context of the publication of information for any kind of general audience. The rearranging of these facts falls under the category of confidentiality.

Truth telling, or remaining healthy one day at a time, does not mean that I must tell all that I know, especially when to do so would be to inflict injury on someone else. And, as I mentioned in Step 9, truth telling is *not* a license for emotional abuse.

Confidentiality is a very important issue in the context of spirituality in that it, like truth telling, is also a contract for trust. In a very real sense, my work as a teacher and pastoral counselor necessarily involves the keeping of secrets. These, however, most often are not the kinds of secrets that make us sick. No, confidential information is shared with me because a person has decided to step out of denial and into the bright light of the truth for his or her life. Confidentiality simply means that I can be trusted *not* to share someone else's secrets. Confidentiality is an act of love and a decision for trust that provides a safe harbor for the truth. It is not the same thing as lying; it is a silent form of the truth. The anecdotes in this book are fundamentally true, but they are so disguised as to remain opaque. Therefore, confidentiality is maintained.

As you have no doubt deduced, this "truth telling" and "truth keeping" business is all very confusing. That is why I have come to regard Step 10 as what I term the "Step of Vigilance." It keeps me on my toes and encourages me daily to remain aware that *every* decision I make is important.

I don't like that fact. I wish very much that such were not the case, but to believe otherwise is just one more way to lie to ourselves, or to slip again beneath the murky surface of denial. To pretend that my everyday, mundane decisions don't make any significant difference is one more attempt to seduce myself into believing that little white lies or "harmless" prevarications don't really fall under the mandate to tell the truth.

In *The Road Less Traveled,* Scott Peck offers the following rules regard-

Step 10: I continue to work on being truthful.

ing telling the truth (which I have paraphrased):

1. Never speak a falsehood.
2. Bear in mind that the act of withholding the truth is always potentially a lie, and that in each instance in which the truth is withheld, a significant moral decision is required.
3. The decision to withhold the truth should never be based on personal needs, such as a need for power, a need to be liked, or a need to protect one's self from challenge.
4. The decision to withhold the truth must always be based entirely upon the needs of the person or people from whom the truth is being withheld.
5. The assessment of another person's needs is an act of responsibility which is so complex that it can only be executed wisely when one operates with genuine love for another.
6. The primary factor in the assessment of another person's needs is the assessment of that person's capacity to utilize the truth for his or own spiritual growth. It should be borne in mind that our tendency is generally to underestimate rather than overestimate this capacity.[3]

Close to two decades ago my father transported my grandfather from the farm to a city hospital, where a series of diagnostic tests were run. I, along with the rest of my family, dreaded hearing the results, which we knew would likely not be positive.

A physician friend of the family and golfing buddy of my father's broke the news to Dad first: "Your father has prostate cancer. We can treat that with hormones and other medications. It is quite likely, though, that his heart disease (which we already knew about) will take him from this life before the cancer kills him."

Some time after delivering that piece of news to my father, the doctor entered my grandfather's hospital room to share with this wonderful old man the truth of his imminent death.

I entered the room, alone, later the afternoon of the day my grandfather had been given his prognosis. As I sat on the corner of this old man's bed, I reached forward and, more by instinct, I suppose, than by any conscious design, I took his callused hand into mine. As I studied his weathered features in search of signs that might guide me to the appropriate word, I remained silent as tears welled in my eyes. I hated saying good-bye to the most loving and the wisest man I had ever known.

Granddaddy sensed my discomfort and spoke for both of us: "You know that doctor was in here this morning."

I nodded as I fought hard against the tears.

"And he is such a fine feller. You know, he just up and told me the truth. He is such a good feller that I kinda hated for him to have to be the one appointed to bring me the bad news. He told it to me with such kindness that I almost didn't even mind hearing what it was he had to say."

I will be forever grateful to that physician for sitting on the corner of my grandfather's bed and delivering to him the truth of his coming death. Such, I suspect, is one of the greatest acts of love that one human being can offer another. Any other way, including a sugar-coated denial of the gravity of the old man's heart disease, would have been nothing short of cruel.

What we say to each other, to ourselves, and to God is important. In fact, it is crucial to our well-being. To lie is to slip once again into the disease that breeds despair quicker than stagnant water gives rise to mosquitoes in a Texas summer. And if you're not from Texas, well, then, trust me when I offer that mosquitoes breed mighty quickly down here.

One day during my second year at the seminary, a kind professor invited me to his office to visit with me about my academic work and about my life in general. He was one of my favorite professors at the time, and I have never encountered a more gentle individual or a more loving human being.

If this academician ever erred with his students, it was on the side of far too much grace. I sensed from the very first moment that I entered one of his classes that he "took me seriously," as we were fond of saying in those days, and that in the agapic sense of the word, the man truly loved me.

Once he had completed his purpose for our brief meeting in his office, he leaned back in his chair, propped his tired feet on his desk, and said something that startled me: "You know, Bob. You will make a fine pastor, someday. You love people, and you're good with them, too. And it is obvious that they love you back."

I nodded in silence, feeling affirmed.

And then he dropped this bomb right in the middle of my lap:

"I never expect to hear, though, that you have written a book."

I am absolutely certain that there was no rancor whatsoever in the man when he offered what proved to me to be a terribly painful statement. But the truth is that this man's assessment of my gifts, not to mention his view of my definite limits, and his "truth" about me, proved to border on devastating.

Step 10: I continue to work on being truthful.

Recently I was on a talk radio program in Austin when the show's host asked me this question regarding my book *On Earth As It Is . . . Discovering God's Grace in the Ordinary:*. "Bob, when did you know that you were a writer?"

I pondered the question and then provided a truncated, though still accurate, answer that had to do, of course, with finally discovering a publisher who was willing to publish my writing.

Driving to a wedding I was scheduled to perform immediately following the interview, I pondered that question and I once again recalled this professor's "loving" assessment of what to him were my obvious limitations. An archaic anger immediately welled deep within me. As I wove my way through the city's Saturday morning traffic, I felt nearly consumed by rage. And to no one else but God and my rearview mirror did I ask these questions out loud: "Who in the hell was that man to think that he possessed the right to define me? Who appointed him God?"

By now I was really seething.

"What right did he have to make such a statement? How much did those words delay my belief in myself? How much did that one statement of his perception weigh upon my already fearful soul?"

By the time I reached the wedding chapel, I had calmed down. I worked Step 2. I focused once again, as I do daily, on what sanity looks like as it is revealed in the life, ministry, and teachings of Jesus Christ. I then began to work Step 3, and I prayed that I might once again muster the courage to turn my life over completely to the will of God. Following that prayer, I decided to forgive the professor and surrender my rage to God.

Then, somewhere in the process, I jumped back to the 1st Step and reminded myself *one more time* that my anger is, in reality, nothing more than a cover for my fear. In truth, I was not so much angry as I was terrified.

"What if he was/is right?" I asked myself.

As I sat alone for a several minutes in the cab of my pickup in the chapel's parking lot, I worked Step 10. It was then that once again I allowed myself permission to know my own truth.

The truth is that I am a writer. This is my fourth book. The third book is a novel which was in search of an agent as this book was being written.

Again, I whispered the truth to myself: I am a writer. For close to seven years I have written a biweekly column on the religion page of the *Austin American-Statesman.*

The truth is that I am a writer. Ten years ago I won first place in a national fiction contest sponsored by *The Other Side* in Philadelphia, and my short story won over more than fifty other stories.

The truth is that, no matter how loving and caring that professor sought to be, he was wrong. The angry, defiant, "unrecovered," and far less than spiritual part of me longed to dedicate this book to that man. The dedication I fantasized would have read something like this: "Dedicated to Dr. John Doe. You sorry bastard! This book is dedicated to you to demonstrate once and for all that you were dead wrong, man!"

To write such a dedication would be to inflict harm on a wonderful, sincere, gifted man who meant me *absolutely* no harm. In fact, he was then, and remains, one of the true saints of the Presbyterian Church.

But the point is this. *He was wrong.* Therefore, a big part of truth telling and what I believe Step 10 is about is the daily decision not to confuse truth with my opinion. If I have learned anything in my more than two decades of ministry, it is to get out of the assessment business. I have no right to evaluate a person's life and to impose limits, if you will, upon someone else's abilities, talent, or whatever. Such is not my province.

Very rarely, even in a court of law, is judgment synonymous with truth. We, of course, are called upon in the context of this difficult existence to make judgments all the time, but very seldom, in my view, are our judgments or evaluations of others the truth.

When I visited counselors and therapists in my search for inner peace, they assessed me and at the end of a fifty-minute session, they handed me a code of numbers, such as 309.28, lifted out of the clinician's "Bible," the Diagnostic Statistical Manual. Such would represent their "judgment" or diagnosis of my "problem."

No human life can begin to be described in five numbers, or even in five billion numbers. We are far too complex for such nonsense. We cannot fit into the pristine categories of clinicians, because we are of God and created in God's image, and God and God's image will never be defined by any human construct.

I once "auditioned" a psychiatrist who immediately told me that I needed to come see him at least three times a week. I recognized right off that I could not afford such a luxury (or was it an agony?); therefore, I rose immediately from my chair in that man's office. I asked him how much I owed him for the few minutes we had spent together in his plush office. He answered in a subdued monotone, sensing, I suppose, that he had lost me as a potential patient.

"One hundred dollars."

As I wrote a check for that amount, I asked him, "What is my DSM III diagnosis?" He seemed surprised by my question, but his answer

Step 10: I continue to work on being truthful.

did not surprise me. "I don't know," he said. "I haven't been with you long enough."

As I drove away from the man's office, the irony of it all broke open for me like the morning sun peeking through a bank of winter clouds. Here this man was certain that I needed to see him *at least* three times a week, and yet he had not developed a diagnosis that he was willing to submit over his signature to an insurance company. My own diagnosis of the situation was that the man strongly believed he stood in need of my dollars. I, of course, never returned to his clutches, er, excuse me, office.

The point is this: our dedication to spiritual growth through Step 10 means that we must remain careful with the truth at all costs. Dietrich Bonhoeffer writes:

> *There is a truth which is of Satan. Its essence is that under the semblance of truth it denies everything that is real. It lives upon hatred of the real and of the world which is created and loved by God. It pretends to be executing the judgment of God....*
>
> *God's truth judges created things out of love, and Satan's truth judges them out of envy and hatred. God's truth has become flesh in the world and is alive in the real, but Satan's truth is the death of all reality.*[4]

What this means is that God's truth is truth and Satan's truth is a lie. It is easier than slipping on ice to slide into Satan's truth, or lies, when I step over a boundary that is not mine to trespass. When I judge anyone's limits or abilities, when I fabricate someone else's destiny, or even when I confuse a string of diagnostic symbols with any accurate picture of that individual's whole life, I am slipping, unwittingly but surely into "Satan's truth."

The good-hearted, genuinely kind, sincere, and affable professor who once told me that he never expected to hear that I had published a book was in effect attempting to love me by making his truth my truth. In effect, what he was saying was, "You are not a writer. Or even worse, you will *never* be a writer." In offering his truth, or what Bonhoeffer might term "Satan's truth," or a lie, and in attempting to love me, he unwittingly confused and ultimately abused me. Such, of course, was not his intent, but it was the outcome of his assessment of me, nevertheless.

There can be no doubt that I have done the same, or even much worse, in my own transactions with people I have professed to love. Be it couched in love or in all-out malice, a lie *always* remains a lie. It may very well look like the truth and even smell like the truth or feel like the truth, but it is still a lie if it is anything *but* the truth.

Spiritually mature people who are willing to live Step 10 courageously are those relatively few among us who also have invested energy, not to mention years, severing the emotional and psychological umbilical cord that has attached them, even bound them, to the expectations and perceptions of their parents. To live an honest, truth-filled life, it is, therefore, incumbent upon each of us to pursue diligently our *own* truth. Such a pursuit is costly in that it requires of us that we let go of long-cherished and sacred lies.

Take, for example, the very first word that I learned to read in the English language: "White." Why of all words did I learn to read this one first? Because I was white, and because I grew up in a culture that taught me that one set of people, my group, could drink at a certain water fountain, use a certain bathroom, and sit in a particular section of the motion picture theater beneath a sign with the word "White" printed on it. Obviously, it was very important for me at the age of five to know the meaning of that emotion-laden word so that I would not dare cross over the lines of race, which, in fact, were nothing more than artificial boundaries keeping a temporary lid on the ancient hatreds that simmered in the culture that reared me.

The other sign read, of course, "Colored." I didn't need to learn that word; all that was needed to get along in the culture was the word that *defined* me more than any other back in the postwar world into which I was born. That word was simply "White."

I learned about the time I was midway through college that the culture had lied to me. (I was a slow study!) Even the wonderful church of my childhood, by its silent acquiescence to racial segregation, lied to me. There were no blacks in the congregation where I worshiped, and I fully believe today that had a black family been courageous enough to seek to join our fellowship back in the '50s, many "good" Christian people in that church would have voted with their feet and taken their money with them.

What I discovered on my own, with no particular support from the culture that reared me, is that racial segregation is an evil entirely predicated upon unfounded fear. No race is, of course, superior to any other. The men and women who taught me for one year of graduate education in a predominantly black university were, I judged, much brighter than I. More than half of the students in my classes, all of whom were black, I perceived to demonstrate a grasp of complex concepts that far exceeded my own.

The culture lied to me about race, and it continues to lie to us about other issues, as well. I suspect it will always be that way in that cultural

Step 10: I continue to work on being truthful.

lies seem as inevitable as frost on a winter pumpkin. Why? The theories are as many as there are theoreticians and theologians. Call it original sin. Call it "cultural inertia." Characterize it is a sick collective unconscious. Term it what you will. The truth remains that we, all of us—and no one is ever exempt from this—must discover our own truth. We must discover the truth of our lives, the truth or the inevitability of our death, the truth of God, and the truth that we are free to make something of this life, or we are free to waste it entirely.

Poet Robert Bly writes of his response after reading the following words of Swiss psychiatrist Alice Miller in *The Drama of the Gifted Child*:

We came as infants, "trailing clouds of glory," arriving from the farthest reaches of the universe, bringing with us appetites well preserved from our mammal intelligence, spontaneities wonderfully preserved from our 150,000 years of tree life, anger well preserved from our 5,000 years of tribal life—in short, with our 360-degree radiance—we offered this gift to our parents. They didn't want it. They wanted a nice little girl or a nice boy. That's the first act of the drama.[5]

His reaction to her insight is as follows: "When I read her book I fell into a depression for three weeks. With so much gone, what can we do? We can construct a personality more acceptable to our parents."[6]

Therefore, part of working Step 10 is, as much as is possible, to step out of and beyond the system of subtle lies the family and the culture at large bestow upon us and to work hard for the rest of our lives to discover what we perceive to be our own truth about reality. Step 10 is returning to the truth, even if I have never known the truth, because I am, in reality, returning to God. And God is the truth. I love the image that Robert Bly employs in his poem of being on Noah's ark and sending out doves, who, of course, old Noah hopes desperately will return with the truth of dry land in the midst of forty days of chaos:

> The dove returns: it found no resting place;
> It was in flight all night above the shaken seas;
> Beneath dark eaves
> The dove shall magnify the tiger's bed;
> Give the dove peace.
> The split-tailed swallow leaves the sill at dawn;
> At dusk, blue swallows shall return.
> On the third day the crow shall fly,
> The crow, the crow, the spider-colored crow,
> The crow shall find new mud to walk upon.[7]

It often feels to me that sending out crows from across the bow of my own ark is what I have been about for a lifetime. In fact, I have come to regard sending out crows as the most fitting image for what I have been about since I discovered the spiritual discipline inherent in these twelve wonderful, difficult Steps. Many times I have sensed myself lost at sea in a giant ark carrying with me a shipload of responsibility. The despair that attends "being lost" is at times close to overwhelming; yet, all that I have known to do is to send out my own kind of crows.

And when the crows return to my personal ark and scrape their muddy feet upon its deck, I examine the mud and discern from its texture, as well as from its very composition, what truth I can squeeze out of each granule. Finally, when a new morning breaks over the bow of my own lost ark, I send out more crows. Little by little, I learn from some crow's muddy deposits upon the deck a truth that possesses the power to guide me home through even the most tempestuous flood.

Frederich Beuchner writes: "Go where your best prayers take you. Unclench the fists of your spirit and take it easy. Breathe deep of the glad air and live one day at a time. Know that you are precious. . . . Know that you can trust God."[8]

That is exactly where this Step leads us—back to where we first began, when we were launched into this journey called life. The beginning point is simultaneously our destiny. In a word, it is called God. In our practice of Step 10, we make a commitment not just to be truthful, but to live the truth and even to become the truth. It is in that commitment that we come to discover more than we ever hoped to find. In a word, it is again what English speakers call God. What more could we possibly need to help us on our long, difficult, and sometimes even dangerous, journey?

References

[1] Frederick Beuchner, *Telling Secrets . . . A Memoir* (San Francisco: Harper, 1991), pp. 10-11.

[2] Thomas Merton, *New Seeds of Contemplation*, pp. 186-187.

[3] M. Scott Peck, *The Road Less Traveled*, pp. 62–63.

[4] Dietrich Bonhoeffer, *Ethics*, p. 366.

[5] Robert Bly, *A Little Hand Book on the Human Shadow* (New York: Harper Collins, 1988) p. 24.

[6] Ibid., p. 25.

[7] Ibid., p. 7 Robert Bly's poem used with permission.

[8] Frederick Beuchner, p. 92.

11

I have been crucified with Christ; it is no longer I who live, but Christ who lives in me; and the life I now live in the flesh I live by faith in the Son of God, who loved me and gave himself for me.

Galatians 2:20 RSV

Step 11: *I seek through prayer and meditation to improve my conscious contact with God, as I understand God, praying only for knowledge of God's will for me and for the power to carry it out.*

Twenty years ago, I interviewed for a job I knew that I didn't really want. The job was to serve as youth minister at the First Presbyterian Church of Dallas.

Much to my surprise, the job was offered. What's even more surprising is that I took it. Even today I don't know why, but the fact is that I did. From the moment I set foot on the grounds of that once-grand old church, I was a major disappointment. Those folks were hard on me, and I was, no doubt, equally hard on them.

When I arrived, the church was installing an imported handmade organ from Germany with a console constructed of mahogany. It was an impressive instrument costing in the neighborhood of a half million dollars. That is a good bit of money even today. Its worth, of course, was

Simple Steps...Costly Choices

much greater twenty years ago.

When you attend a seminary that requires that you dedicate yourself to the reading of the likes of Amos and Hosea in the original Hebrew, it is more than a little difficult—at least it was for me—to appreciate an investment of a half million dollars in a musical instrument. As many as fifty men, women, and children were knocking at that church's door every day of the week begging for food, and these folks in downtown Dallas were "investing in the future," as some termed it, by purchasing a handmade half-million-dollar organ.

The church had been erected on the corner of Wood and Harwood Streets in downtown Dallas in 1913, and for the whole of its existence it had not ever, as far as I could determine from longtime members, opened its doors to feed the hungry of its community. Church members' collective response to "urban blight," as many termed it, was to worry no small amount about their declining membership and then turn around and order one elegant musical instrument so that they might attract the kind of members who would sustain the church.

The story is long, involved, and not in any way germane to the purposes of this book, but suffice it to say that six months after my arrival, I joined others in leading that congregation in launching a ministry of compassion and daily sustenance for the homeless with nine hundred dollars squeezed from the church budget. This new program, which evolved into a daily soup kitchen, was dubbed "the Stewpot" because the very first meal was poured from a can of vegetable beef stew that was then heated in a big pot.

For as long as I live, I will never forget the first morning of that ministry. Those in the congregation who demonstrated a certain recalcitrance bore the name of "legion." They fumed and fussed and soon enough, they began to maneuver behind the scenes and within the body politic.

On the very first day my friend and Stewpot cofounder, the Reverend Jack L. Moore, and I were informed in polite whispers and with the kinds of "suggestions" that still send chills climbing up my spine, one vertebra at a time, *not* to use any of the church's tables and chairs in this new ministry. One woman, who later became one of the program's most ardent supporters, said to me, "I will not have bums and winos sitting on our good church chairs." (Soon thereafter the church provided a comfortable dining hall, tables and chairs.)

Therefore, Jack, a couple of volunteers, and I opened our soup kitchen on a raw, rainy, blustery, late October morning with no tables and chairs to offer our bedraggled brothers and sisters in Christ.

I stacked the paper bowls, plastic spoons, napkins, and paper cups on

Step 11: I seek God's will and pray for courage.

the floor and pulled open the door on the east side of the church. All of us were a bit tense, I suspect, because none of us had ever attempted this kind of intimacy with desperation. No doubt, all of us wondered if these folks would behave and remain, at the very least, civil.

The wind blew through the door before the first homeless man set foot in the church, and that October wind seemed to delight in playing havoc with the paper bowls, spoons, and so forth that were stacked upon the floor. I immediately began to chase after the paper and plastic items, and one of the volunteers turned to me and whispered a word I will never forget: "Pentecost! Pentecost!"

I instinctively argued, "No, Pentecost is in summer, not October!" He grinned and said, "No, it is the first time that the Spirit of God has blown through this old church in years."

As I reclaimed the paper and plastic goods from the floor, I turned to experience what for me became a mystical moment. There was nothing spooky or eerie in the moment, and no natural laws were broken, or even bent. It was as though for a moment, I knew in my heart of hearts that what we were about in that austere, inhospitable hallway, where fear had disallowed the use of tables and chairs, was God. Suddenly in the dark, cold hallway a light formed that could not be seen or described but could only be felt and known.

In that moment, even as a terrified, diseased man of twenty-eight, I knew without a shred of doubt that we were in the presence of holiness and that, somehow, this ministry of feeding the desperate would last beyond all gloomy predictions and would stretch us as a people far beyond any boundary marked by fear.

Today, that same small effort is housed in a three-story building and offers food, clothing, medical attention, and love to the desperate of downtown Dallas. I deserve no credit whatsoever for opening that now somewhat famous soup kitchen because I was, at the time, nothing more than a frightened young man joining others in simply doing the right thing, that is, God's thing, at precisely the right time.

Ten years later, I willingly left that congregation following a mild, but in my perception, dramatic shift in the church's theological and programmatic investment that culminated in the calling to the office of senior pastor a gifted young man. For a myriad of reasons, I elected not to work with him.

Twenty years after the founding of the Stewpot, my friend Andy, the octogenarian saint whom I mentioned in a previous chapter, asked if he could share lunch with me at my Hill Country writing retreat. I sensed that he very much wanted to offer to me a word that he considered important.

He looked at me in silence at first and then said, "Bob, you disturbed those people up there in Dallas. You disturbed them badly. They will never be the same for it. Today they are even sponsoring a ministry to prisoners in the state penitentiary."

I nodded in full agreement with Andy's assertion that I had certainly disturbed those folks. The truth is that I did bother them so much that many of them, but certainly not all, made it terribly uncomfortable, and later impossible, for me to remain connected to their fellowship. I could feel the tears welling in my eyes once again, as they have many times over the years, and I said, "Andy, those folks were mighty hard on me." He nodded, and a new silence fell between us like a fog that arrives to blanket a winter's night.

But twenty years ago, in the founding of a soup kitchen, I knew, for the first and, perhaps, only time in my life, that what I was about was entirely of God and had nothing to do with my ego or my narcissism or my obsessions or my compulsions or my desperate need to be recognized. The moment was simply of God. Therefore, it was right.

Step 11 is about centering myself so firmly, so deeply, in the faith that I can again enjoy a perhaps similar sense that what I am about in this life is right. As Step 11 suggests, the key to any such sense lies in contemplation, meditation, and prayer for the discernment of God's will in my life.

What, then, is God's will? I have been certain only once in my life about that, and since that October morning in 1975, I've never again been fully certain. But I am quite willing to share with you what I believe that God's will is *not*.

First of all, God's will is *never* capricious. It cannot be read in the stars, or discovered in a pack of tarot cards, or revealed in some crystal ball, or picked up like a gaudy trinket at the base of some new-age pyramid. God's will is to be found in one place, and in one place only—in God. The prophet Micah (6:8) tells us that God's will, or what God requires of us, is that we "do justice, love kindness and walk humbly with [our] God."

I figure that old Micah is as good a place as any to begin to attempt to figure out God's will for our lives, and I tend to view his three points—justice, kindness, and humility—as three sturdy fence poles where I can string some barbed wire pretty tight and make a cozy pen for myself. As long as I am living within the boundaries of that tight-strung fence I can be pretty sure, but, of course, never certain, that I am walking about somewhere in the vicinity of God's will for my life.

Frankly, I don't cotton much to this approach in that it tends to fence

Step 11: I seek God's will and pray for courage.

me in (the pun is definitely intended!). I prefer a spontaneous approach to any step that smacks of the constraints imposed by "Christian neo-legalism." But I also don't believe that I can just sit back and contemplate God's will without first being informed about God through what I claimed in my ordination vows to be the norm of my faith and practice, namely, the Bible.

It is when I study the Scriptures that I begin to see that God's will is consistently present in the lives of biblical figures as a distinct, unequivocal call to courage. An ancient Hebrew hears a voice calling to him out of a bush not consumed by fire to return to a land where he is wanted for murder so that he might stand face-to-face with a king. He balks, of course, and makes up some lame excuse about being inadequate to the task.

Another fellow is instructed to travel to a particular city, and he sprints in the opposite direction and ends up in the belly of one big fish. A third, this one a fisherman, follows Jesus through all manner of adventures and then, when push comes to shove, he informs a woman at a campfire that he never even heard of the carpenter from Galilee.

If I am sure of anything it is this: doing God's will demands courage. And so does working Step 11. Therefore, I don't know how to tell anyone *how* to accomplish Step 11 except to say, do exactly what it invites you to do: God's will!

But I will readily offer to you that we have a model of what it means to do God's will. His name, of course, is Jesus. Just as he is the model for what it means to be sane, or spiritually mature, he is also the model for what it means to do God's will. Therefore, as I mentioned in another chapter, doing the will of God and being sane are, for me, one and the same. Founding a soup kitchen in the basement of a once-elegant downtown church was probably, in purely political and human terms, more than a little unwise. In spiritual terms, however, I contend that, for at least one time in my life I was certain, without a doubt, that I was about God's will and was, therefore, right. I have no doubt whatsoever that in that defining moment I knew precisely what Jesus would have done had he answered the knocks on our door some fifty times a day to find people shivering in the cold and sweltering in the summer heat as they searched for food. He, too, would have turned his back on a half-million-dollar organ so that he might claim the homeless as brothers and sisters. Then he would have fed them.

Many well-intentioned folks, from Sunday school teachers to seminary professors, have striven to convince me that the Holy Spirit is somehow "contagious," like some kind of heaven-sent virus. It is as though these folks honestly believe, and would have me believe, that the Spirit of God can be "caught," and once we have caught this spirit, then in most every ethical dilemma, we will know precisely what to do.

Aha! we want to exclaim when we encounter such logic. If such is true, then all we ever need to do is "catch the spirit" in each difficult situation we face. Once we catch the spirit, we will somehow know what God would have us do.

I wish it was that simple. The concept of "catching" the spirit or of relying upon some simple criterion question such as "What would Jesus do?" for my ethical behavior does, I suspect, help in some situations. But even a reliance upon the spirit or asking what Jesus would do cannot always be counted upon to provide me with the rock-solid answer I need. The inhospitable, raw fact is that I will not and cannot possibly know what Jesus would do in every one of the problem situations life hands me. And more times than not, I cannot seem to locate the spirit of Jesus as I wander about in the fog of my own confusion, denial, and suffering.

This difficulty is very human, I suspect, and it is the reason, I further posit, that Step 11 encourages each of us to pray and to contemplate and then to plow through our moral issues with courage.

Prayer for me is not easy. But even with that acknowledgment I confess that Jesus remains the model for me, not as some legalistic prefiguring of what I should do, but rather as the living example of how it is that I make my prayer.

It is no accident, I believe, that the fundamental hub of the prayer Jesus taught us—"thy will be done"—serves as the predicate for Step 11. Such must be our prayer if we are to remain healthy, sober, and on the path to our own spiritual maturity. Even if we don't know what it all means and implies, these words remain our best hope for sobriety.

Almost daily, for one entire year I sat alone in a Presbyterian sanctuary in downtown Austin offering those words to God over and over and over again. "Thy will be done." Then thoughts, cognates, if you will, would suddenly flood into my awareness and interrupt my concentration. Almost invariably, those thoughts would be attached to a suffocating fear. Usually, they sounded something like this: "There is really no one there to listen. God doesn't hear this kind of useless whining. Buck up, be a man, take charge, and quit your sniveling. After all, your many critics are right. You are nothing but a failure, a spiritual 'wannabe.' In truth you are nothing but a miserable failure, both as a minister and as a human being."

I would start over with the words Jesus taught us to pray, and then it would happen. In every season of that year, rain, shine, winter, or sum-

Step 11: I seek God's will and pray for courage.

mer, the high-pitched sanctuary roof would shift, groan, moan, and then offer a sigh. And the apostle Paul's words would return to me as a small voice whispering with all gentleness that I, too, did "not pray as I should, but that the spirit of God intercedes for me with sighs too deep for words."[1]

Somehow, I knew that my prayers mattered, that I was heard, and that it was also very true that I didn't know how to pray, except by faith. I do believe that there is one, however, who does intercede for me with sighs that run deeper into the human soul than words can ever find.

All of this is to suggest that Step 11 is not the determination of some "correct" way to pray; rather, it is simply an invitation to pray the way Jesus did and to permit God to take responsibility for the rest.

Apparently, there is a revolution of sorts going on in this culture, and many folks are seeking the same kind of answers that I sought in that beautiful Presbyterian sanctuary, and that I am still seeking, regarding what it means to pray and, even more, what it means to do the will of God.

In December of 1992, *U.S. News and World Report* offered the following data: "There is a hunger these days, a gnawing dissatisfaction with the answers provided by materialism and scientific progress, a craving for an inner life. Increasingly, Americans are looking for solutions that speak to the spirit as well as to the psyche." My own impressions informed me that such was the case long before I ever bumped into these words. Other weekly periodicals and daily newspapers carry much the same report.

What is fascinating to me is that while, in the "respectable" churches of our mainline denominations in this culture, we worry about our declining membership, the 12-Step recovery movement is growing by leaps and bounds. Each year more new people seem to gravitate to church basements on Monday or Wednesday evenings to work the 12 Steps of recovery than visitors or prospective members show up in our stained glass–decorated sanctuaries on Sunday morning to worship.

What does this phenomenon mean? I don't know for certain, but I suspect that it has to do with the fact that these 12 Steps call people to a spiritual discipline that puts them in contact with God in such a paradoxical way that their lives work. Of course, to do that they must first give up the notion that they know how to make their lives work.

Most traditional, "respectable," mainline churches are still locked into, at best, the religious and cultural paradigms of the immediate postwar era, and they attempt to spoon-feed God to folks without calling them to any kind of serious discipline. I suppose that in the mainline church, we are so hog-tied to the survival of our institutions and the dollars we need to keep their doors open that we quite naturally tend to equate discipline with something offensive. The truth is that we in the "respectable" churches of this culture are often locked into a chronic fear of offending anyone. Our fear is that if we suggest, much less require, discipline, folks might take their money and walk.

There are, of course, institutional exceptions to our attachment to the old paradigms. In fact, I am privileged to serve such an institution at the present time. One young woman in this church, which, by the way, is growing at the rate of about one hundred new members per month, once described Riverbend Church as "Our Lady of Recovery." That is a valid description, I think. And yet, we of Riverbend Church, too, could do a much better job of requiring of ourselves and of each other more spiritual discipline and mutual accountability.

Step 11 does not endorse or bless any particular theology or practice or form of prayer in the religious institutions of this culture. This is simply a courageous step into the spiritual disciplines of prayer and contemplation, when we ask God only to reveal to us his will for our lives and also to grant to us the power to carry out that will.

All of this is to say that if you seek to work Step 11, all you need is the willingness to enter into contemplation and prayer so that you might discern God's will for your life. And even if you fail to discern God's will, just as I did following a full year of prayer every morning in that splendid Presbyterian sanctuary, you may then conclude your prayer with the request that you might have the power to carry out God's will.

Now wait a minute, you will likely interject here. How can I ask for the power to carry something out when I don't know what it is that I am supposed to carry out? Isn't that like asking a fullback to carry the ball up the middle even when he doesn't know the play?

Not exactly. Thankfully, most analogs break down and eventually melt in the heat generated by rigorous inspection. First, this is not some game. This is the most precious gift you will ever be given—your very life. Second, God is not and never will be a coach. God will be at times a patient shepherd, perhaps, but God will never be a screaming, whistle-blowing, demanding, punitive, sometimes loving, temperamental coach.

What I learned in my year of depression, confusion, and terror as I prayed alone in the Presbyterian sanctuary is that, even if I don't discern God's will, I can, and in the context of Step 11, I *must*, request of God the power to carry out precisely what it is that I don't even understand.

Remember, in my own life there has only been one moment when I was absolutely sure that I was right. In that one shining moment, there was no ambivalence. Beyond the narrow boundaries of that episode, how-

Step 11: I seek God's will and pray for courage.

ever, I have, like most everyone else, remained confused, baffled, bewildered, and dwelling somewhere between scared and terrified.

So when I ask God to grant me the power to carry out God's will, even when I no more discern it than a jackass can be expected to read the morning headlines, how do I demonstrate to myself, as well as to God, that I am carrying out the very will that I fail to understand?

My experience with Step 11 has taught me that the only answer that makes any real sense is a return to Paul's first descriptor for love, namely, patience. Therefore, for a full year, one day at a time, in working Step 11, all that I could come up with was that, in being patient, what I was meant to learn was something valuable from the experience.

I am now convinced that through the process of my asking God for the power to carry out what it was that I did not even begin to understand, God was teaching me to trust God. This remains today a lesson in which I stand in sore need of further instruction.

My father once tossed me a pearl I've never forgotten. He advised me to follow a stream if I ever got lost in the mountains. A stream, he said, would lead, in time, to a river, and a river would eventually flow toward some kind of place, meaning civilization, where I might find the help I needed. I've embraced that particular truth for years, and I employ it far more often today in a spiritual context than as a tool for any kind of outdoor survival. In my confusion, and while I prayed earnestly for that year, I also learned to follow the metaphorical stream that flows always toward its own destiny. Meditation, or what some term "contemplation," is the name of that stream.

As a narrative footnote of sorts here, I need to point out that for me, though certainly not for everyone, the terms "meditation" and "contemplation" are synonyms that I employ interchangeably in the remainder of this chapter. Neither of them is, in my mind, synonymous with prayer.

It is curious to me, and, in retrospect, not all that surprising that as a youth growing up in the institutional church, and even as a seminary student, never once was I encouraged to meditate. Oh yes, I was invited and even taught in the church to pray, but never was I offered a course in meditation.

One spring afternoon in the late sixties I was walking past the plaza area on the campus of the University of Texas, which lies adjacent to the theological seminary where I studied at the time. On that plaza area, the West Mall, I encountered a young woman sitting with her legs crossed, knees pointed to the outside, and with her hands resting, palms up, on her knees. Her eyes remained closed and she seemed to be uttering the same words over and over again.

I was immediately fascinated and being what I term a "redneck in remission," I was also more than a little perplexed. I'd never witnessed anything like it. Her behavior struck me as rather odd and, because it didn't fit neatly into my quaint paradigms for the kind of institutionalized spirituality I was learning in the seminary and had embraced in the church of my upbringing, I rejected the woman's behavior as simply "weird."

Of course, what I witnessed on that spring afternoon was the act of meditation. This is not the only form that it can assume, and what I saw was, perhaps, not "Christian," but it was a form of meditation, nevertheless.

For me, meditation has become, since I first bumped into it at Caesar's university, my metaphorical stream that flows to the river that delivers me to the source of all help. More simply put, I have come to regard the meditation, or contemplation, that is called for in Step 11 as my preface to prayer. Meditation precedes prayer but is not to be confused with it. So what is the difference between prayer and meditation?

Prayer is a conscious conversation with God. In our most efficacious prayers, I believe that we emulate a skilled counselor in that we listen far more than we share. But whatever the dynamic or the pace of the transaction in the prayer, prayer is still a conscious transaction or, if you will, a conversation with God.

Meditation, however, is something quite different. It is the emptying of my ego-awareness so that I can calm myself sufficiently to enter into a "state" of prayer. It is, then, an appeal to the unconscious for wisdom, information, feelings, or any kind of raw data. It is not the seeking of conscious contact with God so much as it is a delving into the mystery of the unconscious. Prayer is the actual seeking of the conscious contact; meditation is the unconscious experience of, or preface to, that conscious contact.

When I go on a prayer walk and hear a bird sing, I am distracted by the beauty in that song. Such an awareness is conscious contact with the bird and the wonderful gift of its song, but it is not to be confused with what occurs in meditation.

Meditation is, by nature, always effortful. It requires discipline, and I have come to believe that the necessary discipline involves emptying myself, purging my cluttered consciousness so that I might, as the ancient psalmist proclaims, "be still and know that I am God."[2] In other words, meditation is to be still and listen for God stirring about in the darkest shadows of my unconscious. It also means paying attention deep inside to God as the ultimate shepherd who bumps, nudges, suggests,

Step 11: I seek God's will and pray for courage.

and gently delivers to my awareness, following the meditative episode, the gifts of grace, or symbols or symptoms to which I must pay attention in the conscious mind if I am to experience the kind of genuine spiritual growth that leads to a lasting inner peace.

I hold Thomas Merton to be the most articulate and prolific contemplative of this century in the context of the Christian faith. He writes of contemplation in these words:

> *Contemplation is the highest expression of man's intellectual and spiritual life. It is that life itself, fully awake, fully active, fully aware that it is alive. It is spiritual wonder. It is spontaneous awe at the sacredness of life, of being. It is gratitude for life, for awareness and for being. It is a vivid realization of the fact that life and being in us proceed from an invisible, transcendent, and infinitely abundant Source. Contemplation is, above all, awareness of the reality of that Source.*[3]

Scott Peck continues: "We contemplatives pay attention not only to our outward experiences but also to our inner voices. Indeed, those of us who are religious believe that God actually often speaks to us through such voices: that they may be revelations. We further believe that a contemplative life-style dramatically increases either the frequency with which God speaks to us or else our capacity to hear her."[4]

How do we stop ourselves in the institutional church from learning, practicing, and teaching this art of meditation? What is our impediment to making contemplation a learned, cherished, and affirmed discipline in the church today in this culture? My suspicion is that we don't emphasize the discipline of meditation as the preface to seeking conscious contact with holiness simply because meditation requires enormous effort.

Contemplation is effortful; therefore, we don't want to do it. If it is something people avoid, then we in the church are not likely to encourage it. We don't encourage it because we, who have connected ourselves to the institution, realize that we are dependent upon the goodwill of our congregations for the survival of that very structure we claim to serve but that, all too often I fear, we have permitted to claim our souls.

Why is it that people by the thousands are lining up to purchase books, audio- and videotapes, and are registering in droves for courses and weekend retreats where they may learn how to meditate? And why is it that many of those same people are asking an ill-equipped, but nevertheless seminary-trained clergy for "spiritual direction" when in my student days I never even heard of spiritual direction, much less was instructed in how to practice it?

The answer to me is simple. People in the recovery movement are, first of all, experiencing prodigious pain. They have come to realize that their lives are not working. These people, and I include myself in their number, have found themselves desperate for something that will work. And they have discovered that these 12 Steps work miracles if they work the Steps.

For me, the traditional church, which is still in the main wed, I fear, to the postwar paradigms of my childhood, is not a place where healing is often mentioned, much less fostered, because, as any 12-Step veteran will tell you, healing is hard work and invariably requires discipline. All too often, and quite unwittingly, the traditional church remains stuck in old, polite, antiseptic paradigms that enable denial, both individual and corporate. The sanctuary becomes a haven from the truth of our individual and corporate sickness. It strikes me as more than a little ironic that in many church buildings across this land the "stuffing" is regularly kicked out of denial every time a 12-Step group meets in the church basement while in that same building denial is coated in piety and a syrupy sentimentality every Sunday morning in the sanctuary.

In short, we in the institutional church don't regularly encourage, much less teach, meditation because it requires effort and, once again, the call to such stretching tends to rub against the complacent hides of our biggest donors.

So what do we do if we arrive at this Step and we recognize that we own no more idea than a hoot owl how to meditate? As the title of this book suggests, the steps to meditation are simple. It is the discipline of keeping meditation at the center of our lives, as the preface to the prayer "thy will be done," that is the difficult part.

My granddaddy taught me in the milking pen that if you will pay attention to the pennies, the dollars will take care of themselves. The following is a penny's worth of instruction on the rudiments of meditation. Again, this is the easy part. The difficulty comes in keeping the commitment to meditate.

First, find an isolated space where you feel comfortable and safe. It's okay to pray while behind the wheel, but I don't recommend tangling up meditation with driving. Both require concentration and attention. So, find a place where you can be alone, and that means *undisturbed.* Allow between fifteen and thirty minutes *daily* to purge the mind through meditation

Sit alone for a moment, listen to your breathing as you begin to breathe deeply, rhythmically. Pay attention to the aches and other complaints your physical body may be sending you. In other words, get in touch

Step 11: I seek God's will and pray for courage.

with your physical being, but do not allow yourself to be long distracted or to become preoccupied with the stress your body is reporting.

Once you sense that you are ready to begin the meditation, focus your eyes on one place, such as a fence post or a knob on a tree trunk, or simply close them. (I prefer to leave my eyes open.) Then begin to say over and over again a very simple Christian "mantra," such as "Thy will be done," or, "God so loved the world."

In the process of saying your mantra and in focusing your eyes on one spot, allow your mind to venture where it will. Eventually it will find the God within you and permit you to purge your mind of all manner of conscious clutter.

You will know when you are done with the meditation. I don't know how it is that we know these things. More than likely, it is God who knows for us. Nevertheless, you will know when you are done. Open your eyes, awaken, stand, stretch, breathe deeply, and then, in keeping with Step 11, ask God to inform you of God's will for your life and respectfully request the power, courage, energy, sustenance, or whatever to carry out that will.

Then sit back and listen. Listen deeply as though you were a parent listening to the innermost yearnings of a frightened son or daughter. Listen with care, gentleness, compassion (which means literally to "suffer with"), and, most of all, with great patience. But whatever you do, listen.

Often you will hear only the wind in the trees, some bird's distant song, a child crying, a horn signaling the return of the school bus. But continue to listen. In time, it will certainly come. I don't know what will be said to you, though I doubt that it will be spoken in your native language, but the Word, as opposed to words, will come to you. You will then know what it is that you are to know.

How will this happen? I don't know, because it is all a mystery. If it were not a mystery, it would not be of God, and if I could figure it out and sell it to the world in a neat, packaged formula, I'd be rich, but you'd be very unwise to trust me. In truth, I'd be packaging nothing more than another worthless bottle of snake oil.

Often we go for months, even years, meditating and asking for God's will before we know it. It requires as much effort as it does faith in God. It also requires a sturdy conviction that what we are up to in investing our time (actually, God's time) and energy in this enterprise is not a waste.

I sat for more than a year in a sanctuary meditating, listening, praying, and asking. I heard nothing more substantive than the roof's creaks and groans. But now I am convinced that it was that "foolish" discipline, when

I did not know what else to do, that provided me with the courage and, much later, the insight to step beyond the boundary of the church of my birth, rearing, and even ordination for an exciting new venture toward spiritual maturity and the most efficacious personal healing I have ever experienced.

Marsha Sinetar provides us with the "practical advantages," if you will, of a contemplative life. The following is my paraphrase of her list of advantages.

First, contemplation affords us the opportunity to reinterpret the self more truthfully in the context of the whole world view: Individuals alter their way of seeing themselves, the way they relate to others, work and what it means to be a part of a of greater community. They know and live out their own values, with or without the approval of others, and they integrate inner and outer aspects of their lives in a consistent manner.

Second, contemplation affords us the ability to manage resources, time, money, community service, etc. creatively and effectively. The individual starts to control the various resources of life rather being at the effect of them.

Third, the contemplative life affords the individual the ability to let go of conventional pressures for achievement, material goods, status symbols in favor of more intrinsically meaningful things, activities and goals. This renunciation encompasses a wide range of attitudes and beliefs and entails a conscious and deliberate denial of things which might fragment or render impotent the newly developing self and bond with Self.

Fourth, the contemplative life affords to us the ability to tolerate more ambiguity, change and not knowing. The individual develops the strength, or skill, of living with fewer guarantees and is able to put up with more insecurity. This is accompanied by growing openness to the true self, to one's own ability to find solutions. And finally, the discipline of contemplation enhances our ability to merge self and other interests. By this she means that the necessary balance between selfish/selfless choices begins to emerge. There is in these (contemplative) people a neat blending of inner/outer realities, a way of gently coming to terms and being receptive to the needs of the environment, or of others, as a high pleasure. The sense of separateness begins to dissolve as this perception/attitude grows.[5]

I could regale you with tales of spiritually mature people who, out of their own adversity, have chosen a life of disciplined meditation and have subsequently grown into modern-day, unheralded saints. There is, for example, the recovering addict who opened two halfway houses in South Dallas, one for men, the other for women, where the 12 Steps are

Step 11: I seek God's will and pray for courage.

a daily regimen, and where carjackers, prostitutes, pimps, pushers, and just plain antisocial characters are today living responsible lives, one day at a time.

Or I could fill you in on the details of my friend the physician, who lost his license for a year because of drug-related charges, but who is now reinstated and donating more than one-third of his income and his weekly billable hours to the desperate. He has chosen daily meditation, prayer, and the 12 Steps over any further self-sabotage and its first cousin, self-pity.

The details of their lives as well as of the lives of the other people I could tell you about are impressive, but they are no more impressive than the details of your life, or the details of the potential that lies buried within you to love yourself in a new way, to love others with greater discipline, and to honor God by making your life a reflection of truth.

To conclude this chapter, I will share with you the story of a woman I met more than a half decade ago. She was standing behind the counter of a Dairy Queen in Fredericksburg, Texas. It had taken me two hours to drive a mere seventy miles in a fog thicker than any veil of moisture that is ever prophesied to visit itself upon the Texas Hill Country. Perhaps London is destined for such frequent wrappings, but the Hill Country is ordinarily exempt from such darkness. I was driving to Mo-Ranch, fifty miles away.

I arrived at the DQ at straight up six-thirty, which was good, in that I was scheduled to preach before a gaggle of about four hundred high school kids at nine. At my thirty-five-mile-per-hour-pace, I was in good shape, though still a bit addled from my battle with the fog.

As I entered the restaurant, the woman surprised me. Her greeting bordered on the mystical, as though she had been waiting for me.

"Well, I see that you made it."

I didn't know how to answer and so I said something like, "Yeah, I did." I, of course, wanted to inquire how it was that she knew I was even coming, but I decided against an investigation I figured might be intrusive.

She said, "Hon, here, have a cup of coffee. It's on the house. You look like you could use it. I hear on the radio that the fog is real bad over by Kerrville."

How could she have possibly known my destination, I wondered, as I thanked her and sipped the cup of coffee she placed in my cold fingers.

Today I have a theory that I didn't own back then: when we work Step 11 and, therefore, seek to make conscious contact through prayer and meditation with God, we are also making some kind of contact with what Jung termed the "collective unconscious." In making contact using prayers of "deliverance" as I negotiated my Toyota down U.S. Highway 290 from Austin to Fredericksburg, I was, quite unwittingly, making unconscious contact with a woman who to me was a perfect stranger at one level, but at another, a sister. Unbeknownst to me, she was in her own morning prayers seeking conscious contact also with God. Unwittingly, she made contact with my prayers and was waiting for me with exactly what I needed precisely when I needed it. She offered me coffee, reassurance, affirmation, an admonition for care, an unsolicited weather forecast, and, most of all, love.

Far-fetched? Maybe. But the more I work Step 11, the more such "coincidences" like this seem to occur in my life. I've heard my colleague Gerald Mann say on numerous occasions, "Coincidences are merely God's way of remaining anonymous." I have no idea where he picked up such a notion, but I like it, and I believe that he is right.

Meditation is effortful. The contemplative life requires more discipline than I want to put out. Prayer, the real listening kind of prayer, is hard work and requires more patience than is natural to me. But like all of the others, Step 11 works, if you work it, and believe me, it is worth the effort.

References

[1] Rom. 8:26 RSV.

[2] Psalm 46:10 RSV.

[3] Thomas Merton, *New Seeds of Contemplation*, p. 1.

[4] M. Scott Peck, *A World Waiting to Be Born*, p. 84.

[5] Marsha Sinetar, pp. 48–50.

12

> *Go home to your friends and tell them how much the Lord has done for you, and how he has had mercy on you.*
>
> Mark 5:19 RSV

Step 12: Through my own spiritual awakening, I carry this message to others, and practice these principles in all my affairs.

What do these 12 Steps mean? For me, they may be categorized, but not explained, in one word—conversion. A second category into which their power fits is beneath the word "mystery." Of course, by its very definition this latter word precludes comprehension.

Once we have worked all of the previous Steps, we have experienced a religious conversion that is as mysterious as it is wonderful. Does this mean that we are now healed? No. It simply means that we have experienced healing. Are we finished? No again. We must work all 12 Steps again and again, every day of our lives, one day at a time, for the remainder of our days.

Is that bad news? No, it is the best possible news, because you and I now have a structure, a plan, for living our lives that places every day in direct, unconscious, and conscious contact with the source of all love and healing.

I've never known such a structure before. Prior to the discovery of the gift of my disease, which, by the way, is the greatest gift I have ever been given, I never knew what it meant to be disciplined in my relationship to God. For most of my life, even my life as an ordained minister in an institutional church, I quite mistakenly equated discipline with workaholism (actually, workaholism is a defense mechanism for fear). I viewed structure as rolling out of bed in the morning and "working" for God until I nearly dropped from exhaustion. The more I lived this way, the deeper the resentments I harbored and the more terrifying the fears I experienced. Until I discovered these 12 Steps, the concept of a spiritual discipline remained for me one terribly confusing issue. Until I stepped into the courtyard of a church minutes after being dismissed, stood beneath the spreading limbs of grand old trees, and proclaimed, "I surrender!" I confess that, at best, God was to me a finely honed construct. Even though I now see that God has been in my life from the very beginning, pounding on the door of my defenses, working almost desperately to get my attention, I refused to let God in. It was I who resisted God; it was never God who resisted me.

According to Thomas Merton, "There exists some point at which I can meet God in a real and experimental contact with His infinite actuality. This is the "place" of God, His sanctuary—it is the point where my contingent being depends upon His love." And in that moment, Merton writes, "God utters me like a word, containing a partial thought of Himself. . . . But if I am true to the concept that God utters in me, if I am true to the thought of Him I was meant to embody, I shall be full of His actuality and find Him everywhere in myself, and find myself in nowhere, I shall be lost in Him: that is, I shall find myself. I shall be 'saved.'"[1]

The God I knew prior to my surrender under the trees was the God of my childhood faith, the God of my maternal grandmother, who served every meal she ever ate in her home beneath a painting of the Last Supper. God was also the God of my seminary training, where I learned, and even more embraced as truth, the ten-dollar words theologians employ to "explain" God to others. And most of all, the God of my life was the God who came to forgive others and to work justice in the world. Such was the God to whom I surrendered under the trees on the morning of one of the deepest disappointments in my nearly fifty years.

I had worked the Steps for years, but until that morning, with my back shoved against the wall, I had never truly surrendered. In my own sick way of thinking, there had never been any real reason to do so. I could always figure a way to wiggle out of the difficulties of this life. But on that morning, following more than a year of prayer, listening, sorrow, disappointment, and even betrayal by people whom I once regarded as friends,

Step 12: I give my life away.

I had no better choice. My alternatives had narrowed down to only two: either trust God completely, and that means to let go; or die, if not physically, then spiritually. And in that moment I heard God "utter me," to borrow from Merton. There was no voice, just the relief, the wonderful life-giving grace that washed over me, and in that moment I knew two truths. One, I was not alone. Two, something much greater than I was now in charge of my life.

Four days later, I was invited to join the staff of one of the most dynamic, grace-centered, healing congregations in the entire country. I was not even of their denomination, but these folks reached out to me and said, "Welcome home."

On my first day in that setting, I walked into my new office, which overlooks the unspoiled scenery of a magnificent bend in the Colorado River, and standing before me was the pastoral staff of this church, my new colleagues, waiting for me, each one offering me a sincere hug and saying to me in both words and embraces, "Welcome home!"

This prodigal son had come home, and I knew that I had nothing whatsoever to do with this homecoming. I was standing in that office only by grace. I can offer with full integrity and without a hint of conscious exaggeration that my first year in this new position has been the most rewarding experience of my career.

All that was required for me to discover the joy that I now live one day at a time was to give up, to turn my life, one part of my ego at a time, over to God, and to trust God.

Malcolm Muggeridge writes, "There is a crack through which a tiny green shoot breaks out to remind us that this life of which we are a part is indestructible, and has its origins and its fulfillment elsewhere."[2] My own disease carried me to the place of believing something very different. In a very real sense, I set up my despair. More accurately, it was the disease in me that set that up, but I must bear the responsibility for harboring the disease.

My attempt to exorcise those cognitive "demons" and the devastating negative emotions they bred was to serve God more, by feeding the hungry, clothing the naked, and taking the homeless into the church. I was successful by any worldly measure in those pursuits, but "success" availed me little more than modest notoriety (my disease had caused me to hope for something grander) and even more heartache. The harder I worked, the sicker I became. The sicker I became, the more my symptoms kicked up, and instead of covering them, or numbing them with drugs and alcohol, like many with this disease do, I pushed and drove myself to achieve even more. When that unbridled striving did nothing to assuage my pain, I tried all the harder and lost myself for years in a cycle of despair that could lead only to the experience of the deep pain that attended being dismissed and, finally, thank God, to surrender.

Today I am so very grateful for this disease. It, more than the church, more than my seminary experiences, more than my two years of clinical training in pastoral counseling and psychotherapy, more than all the books I've read, more than the eminent theologians I've listened to over the years, more than my friends, has brought me to the place in my life where I have experienced firsthand God's healing power of grace.

In his award-winning book, *Brother to a Dragonfly,* Will Campbell writes of conversion in these words: "Conversion is at once a joyous and painful experience."[3] The turning point for Campbell was the moment he developed, in the wake of the murder of a young seminarian who had come to Mississippi to register blacks to vote, the one-sentence definition of Christianity we talked about in an earlier chapter: "We're all bastards, but God loves us anyway."[4] In the sense in which Campbell employs the word and in which I borrow it for this book—as "southern" for sinner—I, too, am a bastard. I've never had any real difficulty knowing and embracing that self-evident fact, but, as mentioned earlier, my problem has always been convincing myself that God really loves me. My problem was that I was attempting to talk myself into the conviction, when true conversion is never a matter of talk; rather, it is a life lived by a whole new set of principles that I am convinced are as sacred, and most likely every bit as inspired, as any word written in the Holy Bible.

Yes, I have experienced a conversion. My life is far from perfect, but it is now filled with a joy that I experience one day at a time. Through it all, I have remained grateful for my disease, for after all, it was my disease that brought me to my knees. No other force in my life that I know anything about, short of the threat of my physical death, could have compelled me to say, "I surrender!"

The truth is that today, and one day at a time, I remain grateful. I am grateful for my family, for those who have always stood by me, for those who pray for me, for my new "family" at Riverbend Church, for the scores of people who supported me emotionally during my crisis, and even for the man who dismissed me. He did what he thought was right, and perhaps he was right. I don't know, and it makes no real difference to God. Because even if it was right or wasn't right from God's perspective, it could be made right, and it was made right.

I am also wise like a serpent and yet I wish to remain as harmless as a dove. Therefore, I love without being naïve. Where folks are not willing to love me, and where they still insist, out of their own uncon-

Step 12: I give my life away.

scious, internal conflicts, upon abusing me, I will not intrude or impose upon their lives in any way. But I do pray for those people, and perhaps, some day, they, too, will come to my door ready to make their amends. I have no power over that, and, for now, I am quite content to love them from a distance.

In that I am a writer, regardless of the opinion of one of my professors more than twenty-five years ago, I decided that the most efficacious way for me to work Step 12 was to write this book. So, what you have been holding in your hands or thumbing through is my personal expression of Step 12. I took two weeks off from work during January of 1995 and lived in relative seclusion in a tiny rock cabin at Presbyterian Mo-Ranch Assembly in the Texas Hill Country. My companion for the duration of these two intensive weeks was a calico cat who came to my door at dusk to scold me for not sharing my daily bread.

During those two weeks I maintained a discipline that permitted me the opportunity to transpose a series of 12 lectures on the 12 Steps I offered at Riverbend Church in the summer of 1994 into this book. I realized about midway through this effort that what I had bitten off to chew in the time allotted was quite daunting. But by God's grace I accomplished, at least to my own satisfaction, what it was I set out to do. Whether or not this book is judged by anyone to be "good," "helpful," or, God help us, "theologically sound," it remains *my* 12th Step.

If it has helped you, I am grateful. If it has confused you, then I have probably done my work well because these Steps baffled me for years as I attempted to work them in the context of a disease that by its very nature is baffling. What I discovered is that working the Steps without having done Step 3 is tantamount to hitting Interstate Highway 35 early in the morning and turning north in the vain hope of arriving in Mexico by noon. It can't be done.

I will say that writing this book has helped me. I have now worked all 12 Steps. So where do I go from here? That's easy enough. I go back to Step 1, or to any other Step I need to work today. I will never be done with these 12 Steps because the disease will never be done with me.

My friend and colleague Dr. Gerald Mann is right. There are 12 million Steps, at least. We work each one at least a million times in our lives. Because I have now written this book, I am farther down the path toward healing and my own spiritual maturity. For that, I can be grateful. But, the truth is, I still have a long way to travel.

One last question I would like to address is the place of the church in our recovery. Many recovering people I know dovetail their recovery programs beautifully with the institutional church where they worship, serve, and continue to learn. In the past several years, I have taught throughout the Southwest in every major denomination. In the course of my travels, I have heard inspiring stories of addicts like me who are now in recovery and who are both nurtured by their church and working their Step 12 by giving their lives away to God through those institutions. To such I say, "Hallelujah!"

I have met others, however, who want nothing to do with the institutional church. They have found their church in their recovery groups or in their friends. And to them I also say, "Hallelujah."

In the last year I discovered my "church" in a fellowship of dedicated believers who march under a banner for one stated purpose: "To be a beacon of God's grace in the world." Actually, I think it was they who found me as much as I who found them, but, the truth is that I have been welcomed home to Riverbend Church, and my first year, as I have written, has been the most rewarding and meaningful in the more than two decades I have given to professional ministry.

My point is this: in the context of my own healing, I have come to believe that our "church" is simply that place on Earth where we discover God's grace. That statement is certainly not profound, but then, nothing that I write is ever intended to be profound.

I will leave you with this story as an appropriate way to conclude my Step 12.

Many years ago, I was attending a meeting of the Presbytery, which is a gathering of Presbyterian ministers and laypeople from all the churches in a particular region. This meeting was being held at the First Presbyterian Church of Tyler, Texas.

I remember being bored at first; later, I became agitated. My agitation quickly moved to sadness as I watched two men fighting over a microphone so that each might offer a passionate, heated, and opposing view in the cause of "winning" some point. It appeared to me, though I am certain that such was not the case, that one or both of them were on the verge of losing control. Their faces were beet red, and in the sanctuary of the stately First Presbyterian Church of Tyler a hush fell that was followed by a tension thicker than the fog that conspired, but failed, to keep me from my destiny in the Hill Country not so long ago.

I rose from the pew in disgust and also in fear (because at the time I was not working these Steps and such outbursts invariably terrified me). I was ashamed to admit it, and would never back then have shared my discomfort with anyone, but such was my truth in those days. Not daring to catch the eye of anyone seated in those pews, I walked quietly to the restroom in a hallway. The last thing I wanted was to share with

Step 12: I give my life away.

anyone, even nonverbally, the ugliness unfolding in the sanctuary before us.

Once in the restroom, I sensed that I was suffocating. I loosened my tie and then decided that I would go for a walk. I abandoned the debate in the sanctuary and walked several blocks until I happened upon a playground, where I braced my still-tense body against a chain-link fence and watched as five black high school–age youth played an intense game of pickup basketball beneath a naked wire hoop.

Two of the bigger boys were playing against three. I totally surprised myself as I yelled, "Hey, that's not fair! Two against three! That is not fair!"

Perhaps my outburst was a reaction to the adrenaline now coursing through my veins as a result of the terror I had experienced in the sanctuary. Perhaps I was unconsciously attempting to vent some energy by taking a chance with these playground athletes, but whatever the genesis of my outburst, I, for some reason, decided to yell at those guys.

The game stopped in mid-dribble. A hush, not dissimilar to the one I had not long ago abandoned in the sanctuary, fell over the playground, and the tallest of the five walked toward me with the basketball tucked under his long right arm.

He studied me like he was some trained livestock auctioneer sizing up his latest purchase. I could tell he was not impressed.

"You play basketball, Mister?" he asked.

"I once did, and I was pretty good at it, too." I answered. And then only because I was still reacting to whatever was inside me driving me toward boldness, I said, "I'm every bit as good as you guys."

The tall young man slammed down the basketball and barked, with a grin now slipping across his beautiful black face, "Prove it!"

I slipped out of my loafers, ripped my dress shirt off my shoulders, and, dressed in socks, pleated suit pants, and a white undershirt, began to play one spirited game of basketball.

We played hard until we could see to play no more on that unlighted playground. At the end of our game (which, by the way, my side won), the tallest young man shuffled toward me and extended his hand and said, "You're bad, man." For the uninitiated, that is playground jive for the fact that in those days I was still pretty good with a basketball. I refused his hand and surprised him by offering him a hug. To my delight, he received it and offered his own affection in return. There I stood on a nameless playground in the center of Tyler, Texas, hugging five wonderful young men whose names I have long since forgotten as the setting sun replaced the day's warmth with inhospitable shadows.

Simple Steps...Costly Choices

That particular day, I discovered the church on a playground rather than in a sanctuary. Countless times, I have found it in a church basement where brothers and sisters gather at noon or in the evening to support each other while together we work these 12 Steps. For ten years and two months I discovered it one day at a time in a soup kitchen where the homeless were fed, clothed, and, most of all, cared for in the name of Jesus Christ. Most recently I have discovered the church on a magnificent bend in God's river in Austin, Texas, beyond the boundaries of the denomination that reared, educated, and ordained me.

My point is this: the church is where you find it. It can be discovered most anywhere that grace is the natural climate. Sometimes it can even be found beneath a tall steeple. I have found it there most recently.

And to the one who has delivered me to sanity, one day at a time, goes the glory. May your experience with these Steps bring you similar joy.

Now that my Step 12 is completed, and this book is done, there is nothing left for me to do but to return to Step 1 and begin all over again. Am I discouraged? Heavens no. Honestly, I'm encouraged and glad, but most of all, I'm profoundly grateful. And all that I know to write as a fitting conclusion as well as an appropriate preface to my new beginning are these words: Hallelujah and amen!

> Bob Lively
> Teacher and Pastoral Counselor in Residence
> Riverbend Church
> 4214 Capital of Texas Highway, North
> Austin, Texas 78746

References

[1] Thomas Merton, *New Seeds of Contemplation*, p. 37.

[2] Malcolm Muggeridge, *Something Beautiful for God* (New York: Ballantine Books, 1971), p. 43.

[3] Will D. Campbell, *Brother to a Dragonfly*, p. 225.

[4] Ibid., p. 221.

Bibliography

Beuchner, Frederick *Telling Secrets...A Memoir*, (San Francisco: Harper, 1991)

Barth, Karl. *The Heidelberg Catechism for Today*, (Richmond, John Knox Press, 1964)

Bly, Robert. *A Little Hand Book on the Human Shadow*, (New York: Harper Collins, 1988)

Bly, Robert; Hillman, James and Meade, Michael eds. *The Rag and Bone Shop of the Heart: Poems for Men*, (New York: Harper Perennial, 1992)

Bonhoeffer, Dietrich. *Ethics*, reprint (New York: Macmillan, 1965)

Bonhoeffer, Dietrich. *The Cost of Discipleship*, reprint (New York: Macmillan, 1972)

Brother Lawrence of the Resurrection, *The Practice of the Presence of God*, trans. Donald Attwater (Springfield, IL.: Templegate, 1974)

Campbell, Will D. *Brother to a Dragonfly*, (New York: Seabury Press, 1979)

Campbell, Will D. *Forty Acres and a Goat: A Memoir*, (Atlanta: Peach Tree Press, 1986)

Capote, Truman. *In Cold Blood*, (New York: Random House, 1965)

Currie, Thomas W. Jr. *The History of Austin Presbyterian Theological Seminary*, (San Antonio: Trinity University Press, 1978)

Frankl, Viktor E. *The Unconscious God*, reprint, (New York: Simon and Shuster, 1975)

Lively, Bob. *On Earth As It Is: Discovering God's Grace in the Ordinary*, (Austin, TX: Publication Designers, 1994)

May, Gerald. *Addiction and Grace*, (New York: Harper and Row, 1988)

Merton, Thomas. *New Seeds of Contemplation*, (New York: New Directions Books, 1961)

Merton, Thomas. *The Sign of Jonas*, (New York: Harcourt Brace Jovanovich, 1953)

Miller, William A. *Your Golden Shadow...Discovering and Fulfilling Your Undeveloped Self*, (San Francisco: Harper and Row, 1989)

Muggeridge, Malcolm. *Something Beautiful for God*, (New York: Ballantine Books, 1971)

O'Connor, Flannery. *The Complete Stories*, (New York: Farrar, Strauss and Giroux, 1971)

Peck, M. Scott. *A World Waiting to be Born*, (New York: Bantam Books, 1993).

Peck, M. Scott. *Further Along the Road Less Traveled*, (New York: Simon and Shuster, 1993)

Peck, M. Scott. *The Road Less Traveled*, (New York: Simon and Schuster, 1978)

Sanford, John A., *Healing and Wholeness*, (New York: Paulist Press, 1977)

Sinetar, Marsha. *Ordinary People as Monks and Mystics: Lifestyles for Self-Discovery*, (New York: Paulist Press, 1986)

Thoreau, Henry David. "*From Walden...Conclusion*", in The Romantic Movement in American Writing, Richard Harter Fogle, ed. (New York: Odyssey Press, 1966)

Tillich, Paul. *The Eternal Now*, (New York: Charles Scribner's Sons, 1963)

Trueblood, Elton. *Abraham Lincoln: Theologian of American Anguish*, (New York: Harper and Row, 1973)

Wright, Lawrence. *Saints and Sinners*, (New York: Knopf, 1993)

Wischman, Lesley. "With Mercy and Sorrow," *The Other Side Magazine*, (May-June, 1990)

Yalom, Irvin, *Existential Psychotherapy*, (New York: Basic Books, 1980)

Ordering Information

To order additional copies of Simple Steps...Costly Choices: A Guide To Inner Peace, send your name and address with a check or money order for:

        $14.95
        <u> 3.00</u> shipping and handling
Total $17.95 (Texas residents add applicable sales tax)

The workbook to Simple Steps...Costly Choices: A Guide To Inner Peace is available for $10.00 plus shipping and handling and the Leader's Guide is available for $5.00 plus shipping and handling. (Texas residents please add applicable sales tax.)

   to: Riverbend Press
          4214 Capital of Texas Hwy.
          Austin, Texas 78746

The author will correspond with readers about the book or specific questions. You may contact the author with your comments by writing:

      Bob Lively
      C/O Riverbend Press
      4214 Capital of Texas Hwy.
      Austin, Texas 78746